GCP
AND
CLINICAL RESEARCH

GCP
AND
CLINICAL RESEARCH

A Managerial Approach

UMESH C. GUPTA

Viva Books

New Delhi | Mumbai | Chennai | Kolkata | Bengaluru | Hyderabad | Kochi | Guwahati

Publisher's note

First Published 2011

Viva Books Private Limited

- 4737/23, Ansari Road, Daryaganj, New Delhi 110 002
  Tel. 42242200, 23258325, 23283121, Email: vivadelhi@vivagroupindia.net
- 76, Service Industries, Shirvane, Sector 1, Nerul, Navi Mumbai 400 706
  Tel. 27721273, 27721274, Email: vivamumbai@vivagroupindia.net
- Jamals Fazal Chambers, 26 Greams Road, Chennai 600 006
  Tel. 28294241, 28290304, Email: vivachennai@vivagroupindia.net
- B-103, Jindal Towers, 21/1A/3 Darga Road, Kolkata 700 017
  Tel. 22816713, Email: vivakolkata@vivagroupindia.net
- 7, GF, Sovereign Park Aptts., 56-58, K. R. Road, Basavanagudi, Bengaluru 560 004
  Tel. 26607409, Email: vivabangalore@vivagroupindia.net
- 101-102, Moghal Marc Apartments, 3-4-637 to 641, Narayanguda, Hyderabad 500 029
  Tel. 27564481, Email: vivahyderabad@vivagroupindia.net
- First Floor, Beevi Towers, SRM Road, Kaloor, Kochi 682 018
  Tel. 0484-2403055, 2403056, Email: vivakochi@vivagroupindia.net
- 232, GNB Road, Beside UCO Bank, Silpukhuri, Guwahati 781 003
  Tel. 0361-2666386, Email: vivaguwahati@vivagroupindia.net

www.vivagroupindia.com

ISBN: 978-81-309-1776-4

Published by Vinod Vasishtha for Viva Books Private Limited, 4737/23 Ansari Road, Daryaganj, New Delhi 110 002.

Printed & bound by Raj Press, R-3, Inderpuri, New Delhi 110 012.

D0000/D1200

To

My Parents and Teachers

Contents

Preface

Clinical research in India is advancing at an unprecedented pace. In the midst of growing number of clinical trials, Good Clinical Practice (GCP) guidelines have become the need of the hour. GCP is a scientific document outlining the regulatory statutes and guidelines to follow and forms the backbone of clinical trials. Whereas, individuals, organizations and institutions involved with clinical trials miss to appreciate the fact that skillful application of GCP becomes difficult without a proper understanding of basic concepts and procedures involved.

One of the important aims of this book is to delineate the essential and complex components of GCP in a way that lends to easy understanding, interpretation and application. The book contains minimum text but has plenty of tables and flowcharts to ensure rapid and clear understanding of concepts and operational workflow by the readers. The book starts and concludes with an opening and a closing inspiring note relevant to the subject matter.

A brief introduction on clinical trials in India is provided to give readers a glimpse of the current scenario and trends in clinical research. Research involving humans from the ancient time to the modern era of highly regulated world are depicted concisely and chronologically. "Clinical Trial Framework" – a significant chapter in the book – explores practical implications of GCP with the help of flowcharts, which outline the important activities involved in clinical trails and further describe the manner in which these activities are interrelated. This approach makes the book interesting and informative as well as quick to comprehend.

A major challenge in carrying out clinical trials in India is in maintaining compliance to both Indian and ICH-GCP and developing a system that can satisfy the requirements of both domestic and international regulations. The major differences between these guidelines are highlighted in a tabular form. In addition, a few common issues and certain miscellaneous concepts have been explained in a seperate chapter.

"Quality, Compliance and Management Issues" is an important addition to the book, which outlines how to establish, implement, control and update quality systems in clinical trials that encompass major challenges of planning and controlling the clinical study project.

I hope this book would definitely serve in bringing out the implications of GCP for the benefit of individuals and organizations involved in the conduct of clinical trials. Readers are expected to make the best use of this book and in turn participate in the movement to advance clinical trial activities in the country.

Author

A Word of Caution

The purpose of this book is to make the readers familiar with GCP guidelines in such a way that readers develop a better understanding of its practical implications in the conduct of clinical trials. In meeting with this objective, the contents of this book are presented as an interpretation of the guidelines, and thus one may not find the book to be identical with typical textbooks that describe ICH-GCP, Indian GCP and Schedule Y.

To derive much use from this book, it is suggested that readers first go through standard literatures in ICH-GCP and Indian GCP guidelines.

The subject matter of this book is the sole interpretation of the author and not a compelling one; however, his knowledge, experience and skills have served to come up with the best possible content. Further, the book does not claim or recommend any change or challenge the standard official laws, regulations and guidelines. If any disparity arises with the text, one is suggested to refer to standard laws, regulations and guidelines, and the content of this book cannot be presented for any kind of legal or judicial proceedings.

Author

An Expression of Gratitude

> At times our own light goes out and is rekindled by a spark from another person. Each of us has cause to think with deep gratitude of those who have lighted the flame within us.
>
> —*Albert Schweitzer*

This book is one of the milestones in my professional journey. I have not travelled in vacuum in this journey so far. There are some people who made this journey less difficult. First of all, I extend special gratitude to Dr. Anupama Ramkumar and Dr. Ranjani Nellore who gave me the inspiration in heading the way and providing constant support.

I would also like to place on record special thanks and heartfelt gratitude to my teachers Dr. Devendra Pathak, Dr. Kamla Pathak, D. Shreedhar, Manthan Janodia, Virendra Ligade, and Ajay Pise for their priceless efforts, I can never return, which made me reach to this position and earn success.

Being in the company of optimistic people always influences one's life in a large way. I would also like to acknowledge those who helped me immensely by giving their encouragement: Dr. Yognidhi, Tejal Vaishnav and Ahmed D. Meeran. I am grateful to Anuj Kapoor for providing his valuable inputs and constant guidance.

This book is the result of blessings, affection and encouragement from my parents. They have always been a source of inspiration and stood by me during the testing times.

The cooperation from Viva Books Private Limited, who kindly agreed to publish this book, is highly appreciated. Without their faith in my work, this book could not have come into existence.

I would once again like to thank and appreciate all those people I mentioned and also those I have failed to mention with a hope that they continue to be the source of inspiration and make me a more content and happier human being.

Author

List of Abbreviations

ADME	Absorption Distribution Metabolism Excretion
ADR	Adverse Drug Reaction
AE	Adverse Event
AIDS	Acquired Immuno-Deficiency Syndrome
ANVISA	Agência Nacional de Vigilância Sanitária
ARA	Applicable Regulatory Authority
ARR	Applicable Regulatory Requirements
ASR	Annual Safety Report
BSA	Body Surface Area
CAGR	Compound Annual Growth Rate
CAPA	Corrective and Preventive Action
CBER	Center for Biologics Evaluation and Research
CD	Cumulative Discontinuations
CDA	Confidentiality Nondisclosure Agreement
CDER	Center for Drug Evaluation and Research
CDR	Cumulative Discontinuation Rate
CE	Cumulative Enrollments
CER	Cumulative Enrollment Rate
CFR	Code of Federal Regulations
CHMP	Committee for Medicinal Products for Human Use
CONSORT	Consolidated Standards of Reporting Trial
CR	Cumulative Retentions
CRA	Clinical Research Associate
CrD	Current Discontinuation
CrDR	Current Discontinuation Rate
CrE	Current Enrollment
CrER	Current Enrollment Rate
CRF	Case Report Form
CRM	Clinical Research Monitor
CRO	Contract/Clinical Research Organization

CRR	Cumulative Retention Rate
CrR	Current Retentions
CrRR	Current Retention Rate
CSR	Clinical Study Reports
CT	Computed Tomography
CTA	Clinical Trial Application
CTD	Common Technical Document
CTM	Clinical Trial Material
CTRD	Clinical Trial Registry Database
CTRI	Clinical Trials Registry-India
CV	Curriculum Vitae
D&C	Drugs and Cosmetics
DCG(I)	Drug Controller General (India)
DGFT	Directorate General of Foreign Trade
DHHS	Department of Health and Human Services (US)
DLT	Dose Limiting Toxicity
DMC	Data Monitoring Committee
DNA	Deoxyribonucleic Acid
DOH	Declaration of Helsinki
DPS	Data Processing System
DSMB	Data and Safety Monitoring Board
DST	Department of Science and Technology
EC	Ethics Committee
ED	Essential Documents
EFPIA	European Federation of Pharmaceutical Industries and Associations
EFTA	The European Free Trade Association
EMEA	European Medicines Agency
ESTRI	Electronic Standards for the Transfer of Regulatory Information and Data
EU	European Union
FDA	US Food and Drug Administration
GCP	Good Clinical Practices
GMP	Good Manufacturing Practices
GOI	Government of India
HHS	Department of Health and Human Services (US)
HIV	Human Immuno-deficiency Virus
IB	Investigator's Brochure
ICD	Informed Consent Document
ICF	Informed Consent Form
ICH	International Conference on Harmonization

ICMR	Indian Council of Medical Research
IDMC	Independent Data Monitoring Committee
IEC	Independent Ethics Committee
IFPMA	International Federation of Pharmaceutical Manufacturers
IND	Investigational New Drug Application
INR	Indian National Rupees
IP	Investigational Product
IRB	Institutional Review Board
ISED	Investigator Specific Essential Documents
ISO	International Organization for Standardization
IST	Investigator-Sponsored Trial
IW	Impartial Witness
JMO	Japanese Maintenance Organisation
JPMA	Japan Pharmaceutical Manufacturers Association
KOL	Key Opinion Leaders
LAR	Legally Acceptable Representative
LP	Lead Programmer
MAD	Multiple Ascending Dose studies
MCC	Medicines Control Agency
MedDRA	Medical Dictionary for Regulatory Activities
MHLW	Ministry of Health, Labour and Welfare, Japan
MHRA	Medicines and Healthcare Products Regulatory Agency
MRI	Magnetic Resonance Imaging
MS	Member Secretary
MTD	Maximum Tolerated Dose
MTP	Medical Termination of Pregnancy
NCE	New Chemical Entity
NCR	No Carbon Required
NDA	New Drug Application
NIH	National Institutes of Health (US)
NIHS	National Institute of Health Sciences of Japan
NIMS	National Institute of Medical Statistics
PD	Pharmacodynamics
PhRMA	Pharmaceutical Research and Manufacturers of America
PI	Principal Investigator
PIS	Patient Information Sheet
PK	Pharmacokinetics
PK-PD	Pharmacokinetics and Pharmacodynamics

PM	Project Manager
PMDA	Pharmaceuticals and Medical Devices Agency of Japan
POC	Proof of Concept
PSSV	Pre Study Site Visit
PSUR	Periodic Safety Update Report
Q&A	Questions and Answers
QA	Quality Assurance
QC	Quality Control
RA	Regulatory Authorities
RCT	Randomized Controlled Trial
r-DNA	Recombinant DNA
RFP	Request for Proposal
SAD	Single Ascending Dose studies
SAE	Serious Adverse Event
SAP	Statistical Analysis Plan
SC	Steering Committee of ICH
SCV	Site Close-out Visit
SEV	Site Evaluation Visit
SIV	Site Initiation Visit
SMV	Site Monitoring Visit
SOP	Standard Operating Procedure
SSED	Sponsor Specific Essential Documents
TCC	Trial Coordinating Committee
TDPS	Trial Data Handling/Processing System
TGA	Therapeutic Goods Administration
TMF	Trial Master File
TOC	Table of Contents
TPD	Therapeutic Products Directorate
TRIPS	Trade-Related Aspects of Intellectual Property Rights
US/USA	United States of America
WHO	World Health Organisation
WHO-SEARO	WHO-South-East Asia Regional Office
WMA	World Medical Association
WTO	World Trade Organization

Opening Note

"GCP is not a wallpaper
To paste over clinical development,
We have to build it into our functional system."

Chapter 1

Introduction to Clinical Research

CLINICAL TRIAL: DEFINITION

A clinical trial is defined as "a systematic study of pharmaceutical products on human subjects (whether patient or non-patient volunteers) in order to discover or verify the clinical, pharmacological (including pharmacodynamics/pharmacokinetics) and/or adverse effects with the objective of determining their safety and/or efficacy". The terms 'clinical trial' and 'clinical study' are synonymous.

A clinical trial is a research study on human volunteers to answer specific health questions. Carefully conducted clinical trials are the best way to find treatments that work for people and improve their health. Clinical trials or clinical studies test a potential treatment in human volunteers to see if it should be approved for use in general population. A treatment could be a drug, a medical device, or biological product, such as a vaccine, blood product or gene therapy. Potential treatments must be first studied in laboratory animals to determine potential toxicity before they can be tried in humans. Treatments having acceptable safety profiles and showing the most promise are then moved into clinical trials.

SIGNIFICANCE OF CLINICAL TRIALS

Clinical trials help improve/advance medical research and treatment available for patients. Most clinical trials are done to see if a new drug or device is safe and effective for people to use. Some clinical trials compare among existing treatments to determine the current and approved treatment called the 'standard treatment'. Sometimes clinical trials are used to study different ways to use a standard treatment effectively and reduce side effects. Clinical trials are also used to learn how to best use a treatment in a different population, such as children, in whom the treatment was not previously tested. Usually clinical trials are an integral part of new drug development and are mandatory before a new drug can be brought into the market.

SPONSOR AND SITE FOR CLINICAL TRIAL

Clinical trials may be sponsored by an organization, such as a pharmaceutical company or a government agency, or an individual, such as a physician or health care provider. The sponsor decides the location/site of trials, which are usually universities, medical centers, clinics, hospitals/medical institutions and government- or industry-funded research sites.

REGULATIONS GOVERNING CLINICAL TRIALS

Clinical trials are required to be conducted in accordance with regulations established by the regional or national regulatory authorities. Following such regulations ensures that participants/subjects who enter into clinical trials are treated as safely as possible and the data/information generated by such clinical trials are reliable and accurate. In India, the regulations or guidelines governing clinical trials are available in Schedule Y (Drugs and Cosmetics Act and Rules), Indian GCP Guidelines and ICMR Code. Globally, the ICH-GCP Guideline and Declaration of Helsinki are widely accepted standards for conducting of clinical trials.

ETHICS COMMITTEE IN CLINICAL TRIALS

An Ethics Committee (EC) is a non-government organization composed of representatives from various areas such as scientific community, medical fraternity and law officials, and works to safeguard the community from unknown risks involved in clinical trials. Ethics committees are often known by different names. For example, IRB (Institutional Review Board) is an EC associated with a health care institution, and IEC (Independent Ethics Committee) is an EC working independent of any institution.

Ethics committees are generally established under recognized bodies such as ICMR or WHO. A clinical trial can be initiated only after the approval from an appropriately constituted ethics committee. Procedures of clinical trials are often reviewed by these ECs.

An IRB review is needed to ensure that the rights and welfare of participants as subjects of research are protected. If participants are found to be at great risk, the IRB can disapprove the research or it may suggest changes to reduce such risks. The IRB also reviews inclusion and exclusion criteria to make sure that participants identified are eligible to take part in the trial. The IRB often supervises recruitments in clinical trials. Moreover, the IRB reviews the informed consent document to ensure that it includes all the information required by law to be provided to research participants, and that it is understandable and appropriate to study participants.

RISKS INVOLVED IN CLINICAL TRIALS

Although 'new' may imply 'better', it is uncertain whether the treatment offers benefit to patients unless proved by clinical research. During the study, some treatments show unpleasant or even serious side effects. Often these are temporary and end when the treatment is stopped, but some side effects may be permanent. Few side effects appear after the study is over. These risks depend on the treatment and health of people participating in the trial. All known risks must be explained to the participants before the trial begins. If new risk information becomes available during the trial, participants must be informed.

All those involved in conducting the trial, including the sponsor, investigator, regulatory authority and ethics committee, take care to control the risks of participants. However, some risk may be unavoidable because of uncertainty inherent in involving new products/treatment. Therefore, one must take a decision to participate in a clinical trial only after a thorough understanding of the processes and risks involved in it.

BENEFITS OF CLINICAL TRIALS

Clinical trials that are well designed and well executed are the best approach for eligible participants to gain access to new treatments before they can be made widely available at health care facilities. Clinical trials thus help the society by contributing to advancing the medical research.

PARTICIPANTS IN CLINICAL TRIALS

Volunteers participate in a clinical trial with different objectives. Some think to help advance medical knowledge. Others have tried all available treatments without success and wish to try the new treatment.

It is also important to test a product on patients with intended disease/condition. Eligibility criteria proposed by researchers thus include criteria for age, sex, type and stage of disease, previous treatment history, and other medical conditions. Some trials involve people with a particular illness or condition, while others seek healthy volunteers. Inclusion or exclusion criteria help identify appropriate participants and exclude those who may be put at risk by participating in the trial.

CONDUCTING A CLINICAL TRIAL

Every clinical trial is carefully designed to answer certain research questions. The trial plan called the 'protocol' maps out what study procedures to follow, by whom, and why. The protocol describes the types of patients to be included, schedules of tests and procedures, drugs, dosages, and length of study, as well as the outcomes to be measured. Each person participating in the study must agree to the rules set out by the protocol.

The trial team often includes doctors, nurses and other health care professionals to assess whether a person is eligible to participate. Persons who are found eligible and who agree to participate are given specific instructions, and then monitored and carefully assessed throughout the trial.

New drug products are often tested to see how they compare to standard treatments or to no treatment. Controlled clinical trials generally involve a 'control' standard. One group of participants is given the 'test' drug or treatment, while the control group is given a standard treatment for illness. This control group provides the basis for assessing the effects of test treatment. In some studies, the control group will receive a 'placebo' instead of an active drug, and these studies are called placebo-controlled trials. However, it is often considered unethical to use placebos, particularly if an effective treatment is available and withholding the treatment (even for a short time) can put the subjects to unreasonable risks. Studies in which the available standard treatment is provided to participants in the control group are often known as active controlled trials.

The treatment each participant receives is often decided by a process called 'randomization' done using the computer. During a clinical trial, randomization assures that treatment selection will be independent of physician's preference. Randomization enables comparisons in health status between groups of patients participating in the trial. Clinical trials that employ both 'control group' and 'randomization' are known as 'randomized controlled trials' (RCTs). These trials are considered best evidence to support a new drug/treatment.

In addition to randomization, a technique known as 'blinding' helps ensure that no bias distort the interpretation of the results. In single-blinding, the participant/subject is uninformed whether the treatment he or she receives is the experimental drug, an established treatment or a placebo. However, the research team should know what drug the participant is receiving. In a double-blind trial, neither the participant nor the research team knows which participants receive the experimental drug.

Under the supervision of expert medical professionals, a protocol-specified treatment is given to the participants, which includes specific tests/investigations to assess the safety and efficacy of the treatment. Observations and related data are recorded for analysis at the end of clinical trial. Sometimes, if required by the study protocol, the patients are followed-up even after the trial to obtain further information on their health status.

AFTER THE COMPLETION OF A CLINICAL TRIAL

After phase I or phase II trial is completed, the researchers carefully analyze the data collected to decide whether to proceed to the next trial or stop testing the treatment because it is not safe or effective. After phase III trial comes to an end, the researchers analyze the results for medical significance.

In most cases, the results of trials are published in medical journals. If the clinical trial was an integral part of a new drug development, the results are reviewed by the concerned regulatory authorities and approval for the new drug/treatment is granted.

TYPES OF CLINICAL TRIALS

In general, clinical trials can be broadly classified into two types.

- Observational studies, where the researchers merely observe the effects of pre-existing factors, such as smoking, on the health of individual research subjects.
- Interventional studies, where the research subjects are given a particular medicine and/or other interventions, such as surgery or radiation therapy, and changes in their health (physical and/or mental and/or physiological) status are measured.

The US National Institutes of Health (NIH) classifies clinical trials into five types:

- **Treatment trials:** These trials are intended to treat the research subjects and to measure the safety and efficacy of the treatment given. These include trials for testing a new drug or a new combination of drugs, or new approaches to surgery or radiation therapy.
- **Prevention trials:** These trials look for better ways to prevent diseases in people or to prevent a disease from returning (relapse or recurrence). These approaches may include medicines, vitamins, vaccines, minerals or lifestyle changes.
- **Diagnostic trials:** These trials aim to find better tests or procedures for diagnosing a particular disease or condition.
- **Screening trials:** These trials look for effective ways to screen certain diseases or conditions in a population.
- **Quality of life:** Quality-of-life trials or supportive care trials explore ways to improve comfort and quality of life for individuals with chronic illnesses.

NEW DRUG DEVELOPMENT PROCESS

New drug development follows a complex pathway which encompasses all activities and processes beginning with drug discovery up to market launch of the product. A complete new drug development process costs approximately $800 million and takes 10–14 years to complete.

In new drug development, clinical trials come into picture after the IND approval has been granted by the appropriate regulatory authorities on the basis of preclinical/animal studies and formulation studies. Clinical development for a new drug includes four phases of clinical investigations with the objectives of assessing the safety and efficacy of the product on human subjects. The first three (I–III) phases are required to be conducted prior to obtaining marketing approval for the product, and the fourth (IV) phase is conducted after obtaining marketing approval to assess safety and efficacy in a large population with different disease combinations. This book deals with the clinical development of a new drug, and the complete drug development process is out of the scope of this book.

CLINICAL DEVELOPMENT OF A NEW DRUG

In the clinical development of a new drug, phases I, II and III have to be conducted before obtaining marketing approval for the new drug. Phase IV trial and post-marketing surveillance are to be conducted after obtaining marketing approval. This book mainly focuses on trial phases required before obtaining marketing approval for the new drug.

Phase I Trials (Human Pharmacology Trials or First in Human Studies)

Phase I trials are often carried out in a small group of healthy volunteers (n = 20–80). The tested range of doses will usually be fractions of the dose found harmful during animal testing and is calculated by the inclusion of acceptable safety factor. These trials are often conducted in an in-patient clinic where the subject can be observed by the full-time staff. The subject is usually observed for several half-lives of the drug.

The primary objectives of phase I trials are usually non-therapeutic and include the estimation of human safety and tolerability, including the maximum tolerated dose (MTD), at both single and multiple dosing schedules and characterization of pharmacokinetics of the drug.

The secondary objectives of phase I trials may include early measurement of drug activity (efficacy) that may add a factor of therapeutic advantage into the primary objectives. Although not a necessity at this stage, it may be appropriate if drug activity is readily measurable on patients with a short duration of drug exposure.

Although phase I trials are usually carried out with healthy volunteers, patients may also be included, especially those with end-stage disease and who lack other treatment options. This exception is often true in oncology (cancer) and HIV drug trials where satisfactory treatment options are unavailable. Furthermore, drugs with significant potential toxicity, e.g. cytotoxic drugs, are usually studied on patients.

As stated above, phase I trials are usually intended to involve one or a combination of the following objectives:

- **Maximum tolerated dose:** To determine the tolerability of the dose range and to determine the nature of adverse reactions that can be expected. These studies include both single- and multi-dose administration.
- **Pharmacokinetics:** It deals with the characterization of drug's absorption, distribution, metabolism and excretion (ADME). These studies are important to be conducted throughout the drug development process because these support drug formulation and dosing recommendations for different age groups.
- **Pharmacodynamics:** Depending on the drug and endpoints studied, pharmacodynamic (PD) studies may be conducted with healthy subjects or in patients with the target disease. If validated indicators of activity and potential efficacy are available, pharmacodynamic data obtained from patients may guide the dosage and dose regimen to be applied in later studies.
- **Early measurement of drug activity:** Measuring the activity or potential therapeutic benefit may be a secondary objective in phase I trials. Although such studies are generally performed in the later phases, it may be appropriate at this early stage to measure drug activity with a short duration of drug exposure on patients.

Types of Phase I Trials

Single Ascending Dose (SAD) Studies

In this type of studies, a small group (cohort) of patients is given a single dose of the drug and observed for a period of time. If they do not show any adverse side effects, and the pharmacokinetic data are roughly in line with predicted safe values, a new group of patients is then given a higher dose. This process is continued until the pre-calculated pharmacokinetic safety levels are reached or intolerable side effects start showing up, at which point the drug is said to have reached the dose limiting toxicity (DLT) and the dose one level below the DLT is considered the maximum tolerated dose (MTD) for the drug.

Multiple Ascending Dose (MAD) Studies

These studies help better understand the PK and PD of multiple doses of the drug. In these studies, a group of patients receives multiple low doses of the drug, and samples of blood and other body fluids are collected at various time points and analyzed. The dose is subsequently escalated for further groups up to a predetermined safety level or until intolerable side effects start showing up. In a similar fashion, the cumulative MTD for the drug is estimated.

Food Effect

These are short trials to investigate differences in the absorption of the drug by the body if food was consumed before the drug is given. These studies are usually run as a crossover study (to avoid within-patient variation) with volunteers being given two identical doses of the drug on different occasions; one while fasting and one after being fed.

Phase II Trials (Therapeutic Exploratory Trials or Proof of Concept)

Phase II trials evaluate the effectiveness of a drug for a particular indication or set of indications in patients under study and to determine the common short-term side effects and risks associated with the drug.

The secondary objectives of phase II studies include assessing the dosing requirements, therapeutic regimens (including concomitant medications) for clinical effectiveness with acceptable adverse effects and to identify the target populations. These objectives are mainly intended to carry out further clinical studies (phase III trials) with more accurate designs. Doses used in phase II are usually less than the highest doses used in phase I.

Phase II trials play an important role in the clinical development of a new drug as efficacy of the drug is measured in these trials to take go-no go decision for further clinical studies. These studies are also called proof-of-concept (POC) studies as the hypothesis of drug efficacy and safety in target patient population is tested. The development of a new drug fails usually during phase II trials when the drug is discovered to not work as hypothesized or have toxic effects.

In phase II studies, the research subjects are usually patients with the disease condition under study and usually conducted on out-patient basis. The number of patients in these trials ranges between 100 and

500. The patients are selected by relatively narrow criteria leading to a relatively homogeneous population.

Phase II trials can still be divided into phase IIa and phase IIb trials where phase IIa trials specifically assess dosing requirements (therapeutic regimen) and phase IIb trials study efficacy (how well the drug works at the prescribed dose).

Phase III Trials (Therapeutic Confirmatory Trials)

Phase III studies are designed to confirm the preliminary evidences accumulated in early clinical studies that a drug is safe and effective for intended indication and recipient population.

The secondary objective of phase III studies is to establish the dose-response relationships (relationships among doses, drug concentration in blood and clinical response) and to assess the use of the drug in wider populations, in different stages of the disease, or the safety and efficacy of the drug in combination with other drugs.

In phase III studies, the research subjects are patients of the targeted disease under investigation. The number of patients ranges between 1000 and 3000 or more. Phase III studies play a pivotal role in the clinical development of a new drug and form the basis of regulatory approval. Phase III trials are the most expensive, time consuming and difficult to design and run.

Phase IV Trials (Post-Marketing Trials)

Post-marketing trials are studies (other than routine surveillance) performed after drug approval for the approved indication(s). These trials may not be considered necessary at the time of new drug approval but may be required by the regulatory authority for optimizing the drug's use. Phase IV trials include drug-drug interaction(s), dose-response or safety studies and trials designed to support use under approved indication(s), e.g. mortality/morbidity studies, epidemiological studies, etc.

CLINICAL TRIALS IN INDIA

Over the last three to four years, major pharmaceutical companies have started to outsource clinical trials to India. About ten years ago there were only one or two companies conducting clinical trials here, but now there are well over 100 players.

Indian industry of contract/clinical research organizations (CROs) offer all the facilities needed to successfully conduct phase I–IV clinical trials. These include allied services such as data management, central lab services and bioavailability bioequivalence services. The total clinical services market is expected to grow to $830 million by 2013 at CAGR of 29%. This phenomenal growth is expected to come.

India presently has a very small share of the global opportunity. The total number of clinical trials in India stood to less than 2% of the global clinical trials in 2007. With all major pharmaceutical/biotech companies and CROs establishing their presence in India, the number of clinical trials in the country is expected to grow several folds in the next five years. The country has been projected to conduct nearly 5% of the global clinical trials by 2012. However, the country has been facing challenges like unethical trials, delay in trial approval, lack of protection of clinical data, and lack of GCP certified sites and investigators.

INDIA – AN IDEAL DESTINATION FOR CLINICAL TRIALS

The following factors play a major role in making India an ideal destination for clinical trials.

(a) Shorter Time Period

Clinical trials may be completed up to 75% faster than in the US or Europe due to the following factors;

- Operational flexibility to manage "crunch" periods.
- Speedy patient recruitment – Recruitment can be 4–5 times faster than in the corresponding centers in Europe and the USA.
- Investigators have much influence over the patients.
- India's urban population is keen to volunteer for trials.
- Good patient compliance and retention.

(b) Speedy Regulatory Approvals

Regulatory approval has become more streamlined and predictable. Fast Track Regulatory approvals may be obtained in 6–8 weeks (Table 1).

Table 1 Typical Timelines for Regulatory Approvals

Regulatory Body	Approval	Time
Drug Controller General of India (DCGI)	Regulatory approval to conduct study in India	• ~ 4 weeks – fast track, US IND/EU CTA available • ~ 16 weeks, no documentation to support successful US IND/EU CTA
Drug Controller General of India (DCGI)	Test license to import trial supplies	~ 2 weeks in addition
Ethics Committee	Local ethics committee approval by site	~ 6-8 weeks in parallel
Total (Parallel Processing)	-	• ~ 6-8 weeks (fast track) • ~ 16 weeks
Directorate General of Foreign Trade (DGFT)	Permission to export blood samples	~ Additional 2-4 weeks

(c) Gene Pool Advantage

- Heterogeneous mix of people
- Vast and diverse diseases and patient population

(d) Large and Faster Growing Talent and Resource Pool

- A very large pool of highly trained nurses, physicians, pharmacy professionals and other technical personnel is available.
- A large pool of IT professionals.
- Motivated, English-speaking investigators are present. The medical system transacts much of its work in English.
- A vast range of professional services is available in global standards, including data entry and verification, statistical analysis, medical writing, software programming and data management.

(e) 30–50% Overall Cost Advantage

- The salaries of professionals are 30% lesser than that of those in the West. Furthermore, costs of getting approval, patient insurance and investments over clinical investigators are lower than that in the US and other developed countries.
- Availability of urban-centric, cost-effective health care system.

(f) Credible Data Quality

- Good compliance with global ethical and regulatory standards such as ISO and ICH-GCP.

- The number of facilities providing GCP standards is increasing. Last but not least, the FDA has begun accepting New Drug Application (NDA) that includes data from Indian trial sites.

(g) Wide Range of Disease Prevalence in India

- Access to a large population of patients with diseases similar as in the tropical and industrialized world – Increasingly the Indian population suffers not merely from infectious diseases but also from maladies that are common in the West such as diabetes, cardiovascular problems and cancer.
- Many patients are 'treatment-naïve' (that is, they have not been treated for this condition before), which helps in assessing the effects of a new drug without overlapping.

(h) Ethics

- Government initiatives aim to strengthen the approval processes of ethics committees.
- Informed consent is of critical importance.

(i) Intellectual Property Protection

After the implementation of product patent regime in 2005 and TRIPS and WTO standards, India is in compliance with and committed to enforce intellectual property protection. In addition to process patents, product patents are also now recognized.

(j) Growth of Clinical Research Benefits Indian Patients

- Study participants have access to biomedical innovation.
- All participants enjoy improved care.
- Overall benefit to health care delivery in the country.
- Injection of resources into local health care system.
- Improvements in the standards of medical practice, including communication, record keeping, evidence-based medicine.
- No exploitation if ICH GCP standards are followed.

(k) Resource Development Initiatives

Various initiatives have been taken and proposed at government, industrial and institutional levels in the direction of opportunities created by clinical trial market in India. These include:

- Investment for education and training (state and private)
- Industry (pharma/CRO)-led internal training
- Development of infrastructure
- Investment in staff development
- Creating a global workplace

CHALLENGES IN INDIA

India is rapidly developing into a global hub for clinical trials. While companies are showing positive attitude towards the possibilities of carrying out high-quality research in India, there are still concerns over its capability to maintain and grow in the sector of clinical research.

- Lack of adequate competent human resources for clinical research
- Inadequacy of personnel with thorough knowledge of local and global regulatory processes and guidelines (FDA/EMEA)
- Limited practical experience in the area of clinical research
- Rising salary expectations of researchers as compared to the Western countries
- Is clinical trial data gathered and processed by international standards? One big issue is the quality of data and the ability of Indian CROs to relay it back for analysis. India needs to focus on developing clinical research infrastrucure comparable with US and EU standards and to follow ICH guidelines.
- Lack of interrelations with investigators and vendors.
- Lack of ethical standards to safeguard the rights of subjects and patients involved in clinical trials.
- Are the subjects of trials sufficiently informed to give consent? Are the IRBs sufficiently competent to review clinical processes or protocols? Recruitment of subjects in India is certainly easier than in the West, but there are issues relating to informed consent, language barrier and financial incentives. Difficulties arise due to poor educational status of patients (difficulty in providing informed consent), language issues, widespread use of traditional herbal medication that could potentially confound trial results, and the limited number of hospitals with properly constituted ethics committees.

Appendix I History of Research in Humans: Genesis of Regulations

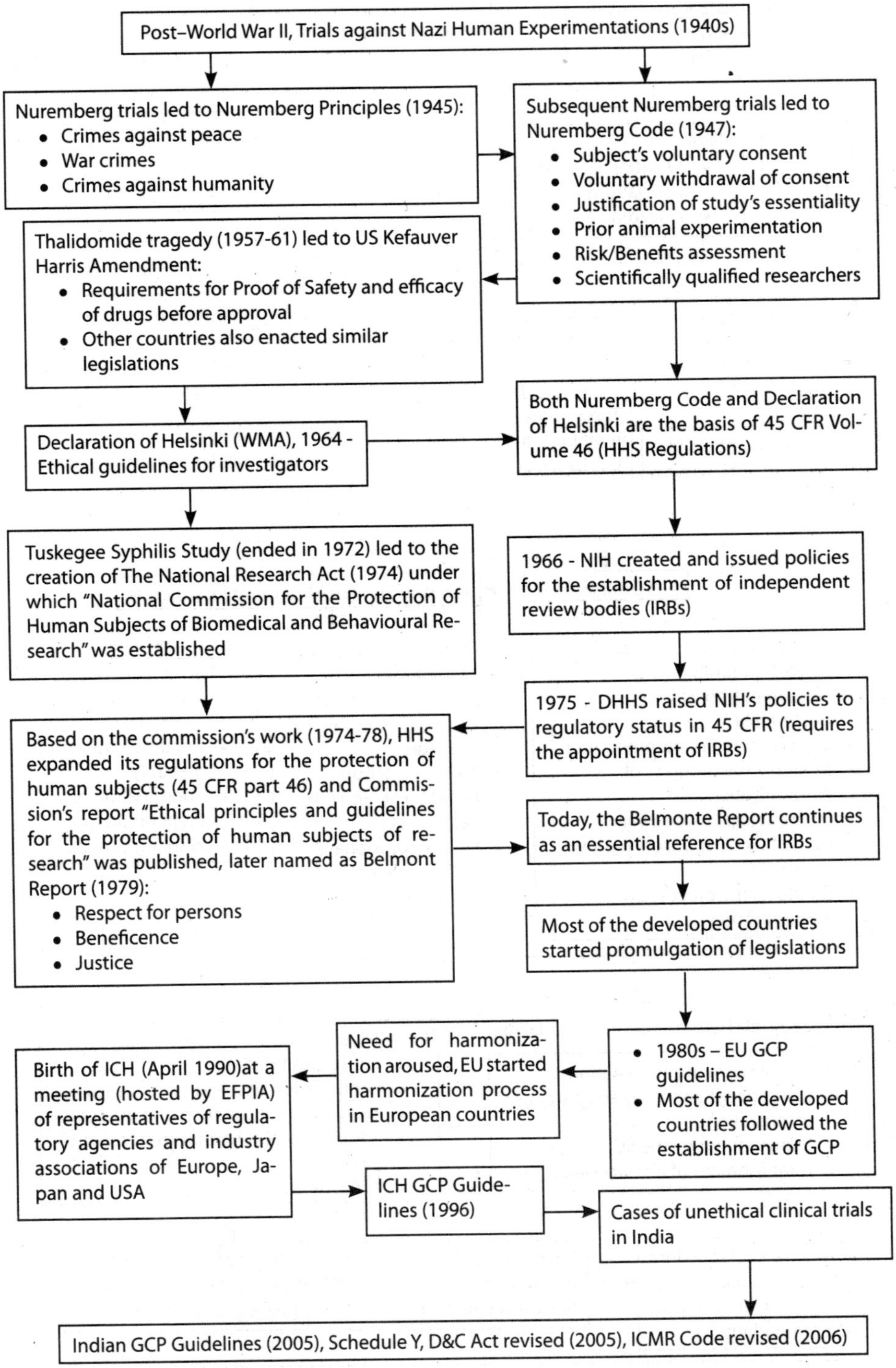

Appendix II International Conference on Hormonization

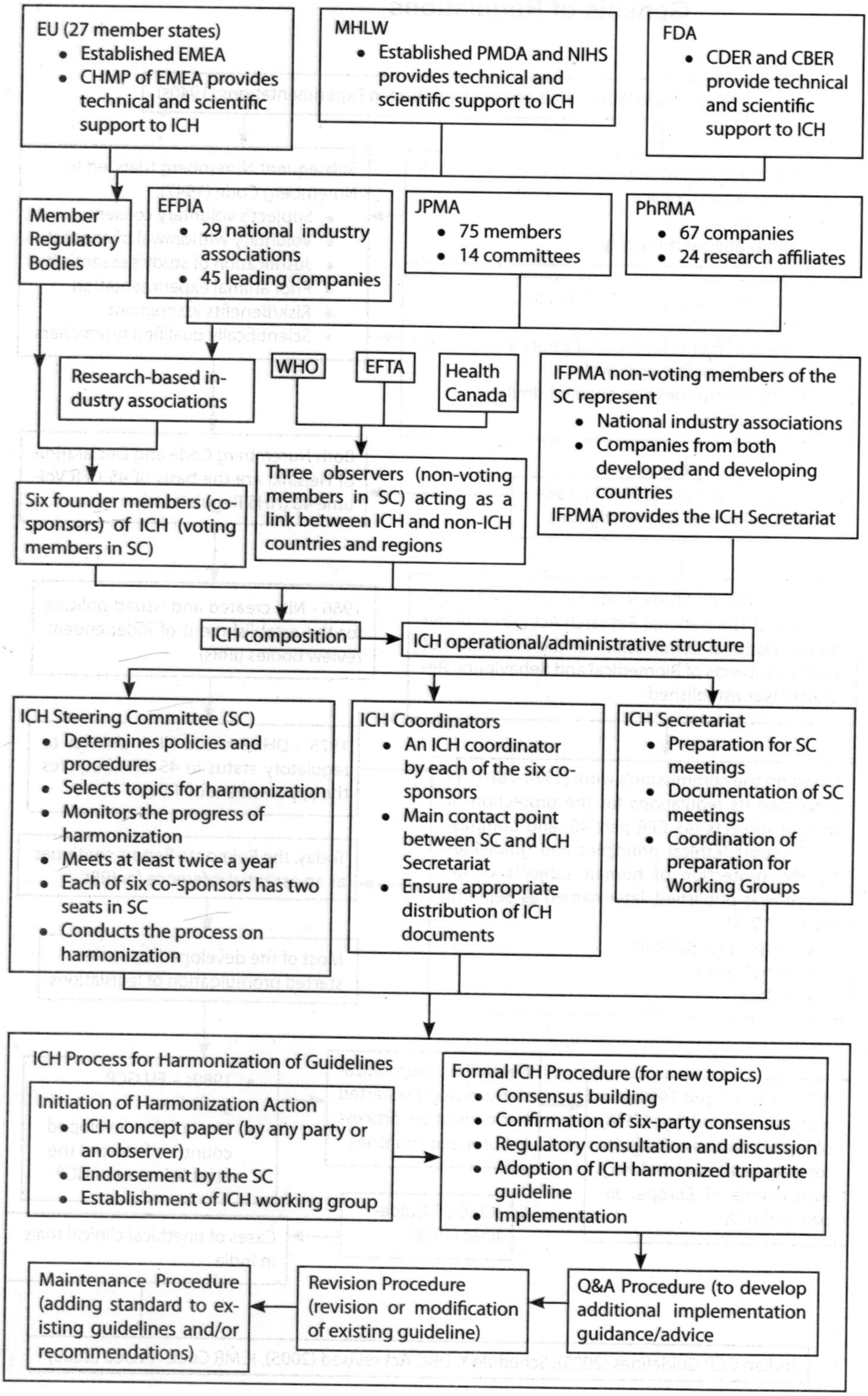

Appendix III ICH Guidelines

Q	S	E	M
"Quality" Topics, i.e., those relating to chemical and pharmaceutical quality assurance (Stability Testing, Impurity Testing, etc.)	"Safety" Topics, i.e., those relating to *in vitro* and *in vivo* pre-clinical studies (Carcinogenicity Testing, Genotoxicity Testing, etc.)	"Efficacy" Topics, i.e., those relating to clinical studies involving human subjects (Dose Response Studies, Good Clinical Practices, etc.)	"Multidisciplinary" Topics, i.e., cross-cutting topics which do not fit uniquely into other categories (MedDRA, ESTRI, M3, CTD, M5)

Appendix IV ICH Efficacy Topics

Code	Topic
Clinical Safety	
E1	The Extent of Population Exposure to Assess Clinical Safety for Drug Intended For Long-Term Treatment of Non-Life-Threatening Conditions
E2A	Clinical Safety Data Management: Definitions and Standards for Expedited Reporting
E2B(R3)	Clinical Safety Data Management: Data Elements for Transmission of Individual Case Safety Reports
E2B–QAs	Implementation Working Group Questions and Answers
E2C(R1)	Clinical Safety Data Management: Periodic Safety Update Reports for Marketed Drugs
E2D	Post-Approval Safety Data Management – Definitions and Standard for Expedited Reporting
E2E	Pharmacovigilance Planning
E2F	Development Safety Update Report
Clinical Study Reports	
E3	Structure and Content of Clinical Study Reports
Dose-Response Studies	
E4	Dose-Response Information to Support Drug Registration
Ethnic Factors	
E5(R1)	Ethnic Factors In the Acceptability of Foreign Clinical Data
E5–QAs	Implementation Working Group Questions and Answers
Good Clinical Practice	
E6(R1)	Guideline for Good Clinical Practice
Clinical Trials	
E7	Studies in Support of Special Populations: Geriatrics
E8	General Considerations for Clinical Trials
E9	Statistical Considerations in the Design of Clinical Trials
E10	Choice of Control Group in Clinical Trials
E11	Clinical Investigation of Medical Products in the Pediatric Population
Guidelines for Clinical Evaluation by Therapeutic Category	
E12	Principles for Clinical Evaluation of New Anti-hypertensive Drugs
Clinical Evaluation	
E14	Clinical Evaluation of QT/QTC Interval Prolongation and Proarrhythmic Potential for Non-Antiarrythmic Drugs
Pharmacogenomics	
E15	Terminology in Pharmacogenomics

Chapter 2

ICH-GCP versus Indian GCP

DIFFERENCES IN GLOSSARY OF TERMS/DEFINITIONS

Terms Described Additionally in ICH-GCP	Terms Described Additionally in Indian GCP
Amendment to the Protocol	Act
Applicable Regulatory Requirement(s)	Clinical Trial (Clinical Study) with definitions of Human/ Clinical Pharmacology trials (Phase I), Exploratory trials (Phase II), Confirmatory trials (Phase III) and Phase IV
Approval (in relation to IRB)	Co-Investigator
Audit Certificate	Escape Treatment
Audit Report	Investigational Labeling
Audit Trail	Monitor
Compliance (in relation to Trials)	Non-Therapeutic Study
Coordinating Committee	Pharmaceutical Product(s)
Direct Access	Principal Investigator
IDMC (DSMB, Monitoring Committee, Data Monitoring Committee)	Raw Data
Institutional Review Board (IRB)	Schedule
Investigator/Institution	Study Product
Interim Clinical Trial/Study Report	Subject Files / Patient Files
Legally Acceptable Representative	Study Management
Monitoring	Validation
Monitoring Report	
Opinion (in relation to IEC)	
Original Medical Record	
Source Documents	
Sponsor-Investigator	
Trial Site	
Unexpected Adverse Drug Reaction	
Vulnerable Subjects	
Well-being (of the Trial Subject)	

ICH-GCP VERSUS INDIAN GCP – A GLIMPSE

(**Note:** Only differences but not similarities are described here.)

Topic	As per Indian GCP	As per ICH-GCP
ICH-GCP has mostly used the term 'trial' whereas Indian GCP has used the term 'study'. One should not confuse with these terms having the same practical meaning		
Principles		
Principles of GCP	12 ethical principles and ICMR ethical guidelines are recommended to follow	13 principles are described
Independent Ethics Committee/Institutional Review Board		
Interim review of trial by IRB/IEC	No specific time has been specified	At least once per year as appropriate to the degree of risks to human subjects
Composition of IRB/IEC	Refer to the section of 'IRB/IEC Composition'	
Decision-making Process	Explained elaborately	Not elaborated separately
Confirmation of IRB/IEC Review	The sponsor shall obtain from the investigator(s) and/or the institutions the particulars about the members of the investigator's/institution's Ethics Committee including their names, addresses, qualifications and experience	The sponsor should obtain from the investigator/institution the name and address of the investigator's/institution's IRB/IEC
Sponsor–Investigator/Institution Agreement		
Agreement between sponsor and investigator	The sponsor and the investigator(s) should sign a copy of the Protocol and the SOPs or an alternative document to confirm their agreement	The sponsor and the investigator/institution should sign the protocol, or an alternative document, to confirm the agreement
Essential Documents		
Description of the requirements of location of documents is given for TMFs of	Investigator/institution, sponsor, CRO and IRB/IEC	Investigator/institution and sponsor
Signed agreements between involved parties	Not part of essential documents	Is part of essential documents
Medical/laboratory/technical procedures/tests • certification or • accreditation or • established quality control and/or external quality assessment or • other validation (where required)	These are not part of essential documents in 'before the trial' section of TMF but required in 'during the trial' section of TMF (information regarding updates is not mentioned)	These are essential documents in 'before the trial' section of TMF and updates of these documents are essential in 'during the trial' section of TMF
Advertisement for subject recruitment (if used)	Recommended to be retained in the files of both investigator and sponsor	Recommended to be retained only in the files of investigator

Contd...

Topic	As per Indian GCP	As per ICH-GCP
Sample of label(s) attached to investigational product container(s)	Recommended to be retained in the files of both investigator and sponsor	Recommended to be retained only in the files of sponsor
Relevant communications other than site visits	Not recommended to be retained in the files of sponsor	Recommended to be retained in the files of both investigator and sponsor
Signed informed consent forms and source documents	Recommended to be retained in the files of both investigator (original) and sponsor (copy)	Recommended only to be retained in the files of investigator
Documentation of CRF corrections	Recommended to be retained as original in the files of investigator and as copy in the files of sponsor	Recommended to be retained as original in the files of sponsor and as copy in the files of investigator
Subject identification code list Subject enrollment log Completed subject identification code list Final report by investigator to IRB/IEC where required, and where applicable, to the regulatory Authorities	Recommended to be retained in the files of both investigator and sponsor	Recommended to be retained only in the files of investigator
Record retention by EC after trial completion	For at least a period of 5 years if it is not possible to maintain the same permanently	For a period of at least 3 years
Record retention by sponsor after trial completion	Three years after the completion of the study or submission of the data to the regulatory authorities whichever is later	Till 2 years after the last marketing approval in the ICH region
Expedited Reporting		
Serious and unexpected ADRs (expedite reporting)	Sponsor should expedite the reporting of all serious and/or unexpected adverse drug reactions	The sponsor should expedite the reporting of all adverse drug reactions (ADRs) that are both serious and unexpected
Recruitment of Special Groups as Trial Subjects		
Pregnant or nursing/ lactating women, children and vulnerables	Additional safeguards/protection regarding recruitment/selection of special groups as research subjects should be considered. These considerations have been described in detail	ICH-GCP does not mention a separate clause for recruitment of such subjects
Impartial Witness		
Presence of impartial witness	As a general rule obtain from each prospective subject a signed form as an evidence of informed consent (written informed consent) preferably witnessed by a person not related to the trial	If a subject is unable to read or if a legally acceptable representative is unable to read, an impartial witness should be present during the entire informed consent discussion

Contd...

Topic	As per Indian GCP	As per ICH-GCP
Essential Information to be Provided to the Subjects		
Essential information to be provided to subjects prior to obtaining informed consent	• Subject's right to prevent use of his/her biological sample (DNA, cell-line, etc.) at any time during the conduct of the research • The foreseeable extent of information on possible current and future uses of the biological material and of the data to be generated from the research and if the material is likely to be used for secondary purposes or would be shared with others, clear mention of the same • Risk of discovery of biologically sensitive information • Publication, if any, including photographs and pedigree charts	These additional elements not specified clearly
Sponsor		
Role of foreign sponsor	Description provided separately	Not specified separately
Record Keeping and Data Handling		
Responsibilities of investigator	Laboratory values with normal reference ranges should always be recorded on a CRF or enclosed with the CRF In the medical records of the patient(s), it should be clearly indicated that the individual is participating in a clinical trial Laboratory values that differ importantly from previous values (in addition to the values out of reference range) must be evaluated and commented upon by the investigator. Data other than that requested by the Protocol may appear on the CRF clearly marked as the additional findings and their significance described by the investigator Units of measurement must always be stated and transformation of units must always be indicated and documented	Separate description of these additional elements not mentioned
Data ownership	Ownership of the data and any transfer of the ownership of data should be documented and intimated to the concerned parties	Any transfer of ownership of data should be reported by sponsor to the appropriate authorities, as required by the applicable regulatory requirements

Contd...

Topic	As per Indian GCP	As per ICH-GCP
Investigational Product(s) Samples		
Retention period for IP samples	No specific time mentioned	To the extent stability permits, samples should be retained either until the analyses of the trial data are complete or as required by the applicable regulatory requirement(s), whichever represents the longer retention period.
Special Concerns		
Clinical trials of vaccines	Description provided	Not mentioned
Clinical trials of contraceptives		
Clinical trials with surgical procedures/ medical devices		
Clinical trials for diagnostic agents/use of radioactive materials and X-rays		
Clinical trials of Herbal Remedies and Medicinal Plants		
Appendices		
Declaration of Helsinki	Provided in Appendix I	Not mentioned
Requirements and guidelines on clinical trials for import and manufacture of new drug	Provided in Appendix II	Not mentioned
	Data requirements for permission of undertaking clinical trial	
	Appendix I to Schedule Y – Data required to be submitted with application for permission to market a new drug	
	Appendix I to Schedule YI – Format for submission of clinical trial reports	
	Appendix III to Schedule Y – Animal toxicity requirements for clinical trials and marketing of a new drug	
	Appendix IV to Schedule Y – Number of animals for long-term toxicity studies	
	Appendix V to Schedule Y – Patient consent form	
	Appendix VI to Schedule Y – Data requirements of fixed dose combinations	
Format for submission of preclinical and clinical data for r-DNA based vaccines, diagnostics and other biologicals	Provided in Appendix III	Not mentioned

IRB/IEC COMPOSITION

<table>
<tr><th>Criteria</th><th>ICH-GCP</th><th>Indian GCP</th><th>ICMR Code</th><th>Schedule Y</th></tr>
<tr><td>Minimum number of members</td><td>It is recommended that the IRB/IEC should include at least five members</td><td>The number of persons in an ethical committee should be kept fairly small (5-7 members) as it should be kept in mind that too large a committee will make it difficult in reaching consensus opinion</td><td rowspan="2">The number of persons in an ethics committee should be kept fairly small (8-12 members)</td><td>An EC should have at least seven (7) members</td></tr>
<tr><td>Maximum number of members</td><td>Not specified clearly</td><td>There is no specific recommendation for a widely acceptable maximum number of persons; however 12-15 is the maximum recommended number</td><td>Not specified clearly</td></tr>
<tr><td>Number of members required for quorum</td><td>An IRB/IEC should make its decisions at announced meetings at which at least a quorum, as stipulated in its written operating procedures, is present</td><td colspan="2">It is generally accepted that a minimum of 5 persons is required to compose/ form a quorum (ICMR – without which a decision regarding the research should not be taken)</td><td>For review of each protocol the quorum of EC should have at least 5 members</td></tr>
<tr><td>Members independent/ outside of the institution</td><td>It is recommended that the IRB/IEC should include at least one member who is independent of the institution/trial site</td><td colspan="2">(ICMR – The IEC should appoint from among its members a Chairman) The Chairperson of the committee should preferably be from outside the institution and not head of the same institution to maintain the independence of the committee</td><td rowspan="2">In any case, the EC must include at least one member who is independent of the institution / trial site.
EC should appoint, from among its members, a Chairperson (who is from outside the institution) and a Member Secretary</td></tr>
<tr><td>Member Secretary</td><td>Not specified clearly</td><td colspan="2">Member Secretary (ICMR – should be from the same Institution) who generally belongs to the same institution should conduct the business of the committee</td></tr>
<tr><td>Members whose primary area of interest is in a non-scientific area</td><td>It is recommended that the IRB/IEC should include at least one member whose primary area of interest is in a nonscientific area</td><td>Members should be a mix of medical/ non-medical, scientific and non-scientific persons including lay public to reflect different viewpoints</td><td></td><td>In any case, the ethics committee must include at least one member whose primary area of interest / specialization is non-scientific</td></tr>
</table>

Contd...

<table>
<tr><th>Criteria</th><th>ICH-GCP</th><th>Indian GCP</th><th>ICMR Code</th><th>Schedule Y</th></tr>
<tr><td rowspan="3">Representation of members</td><td rowspan="3">Not specified clearly</td><td colspan="3">Apart from chairman and member secretary other members should be a mix of medical/non-medical, scientific and non-scientific persons, including lay public (ICMR – persons), to reflect the different viewpoints (ICMR – points of view)</td></tr>
<tr><td>There should be adequate representation of age, gender, community etc. to safeguard the interests and welfare of all sections of the community/society</td><td>EC can have as its members, individuals from other institutions or communities with adequate representation of age and gender to safeguard the interests and welfare of all sections of the community/society</td><td rowspan="2">There should be appropriate gender representation</td></tr>
<tr><td colspan="2">Members should be aware of local, social and cultural norms, as this is the most important social control mechanism</td></tr>
<tr><td>Voting members for providing opinion on a trial-related matters</td><td>• Only those IRB/IEC members who are independent of the investigator and the sponsor of the trial should vote/provide opinion on a trial-related matter
• Only members who participate in the IRB/IEC review and discussion should vote/provide their opinion and/or advise
• The investigator may provide information on any aspect of the trial, but should not participate in the deliberations of the IRB/IEC or in the vote/opinion of the IRB/IEC.</td><td>Not specified clearly, however if necessary, the applicant/investigator may be invited to present the protocol or offer clarifications in the meeting</td><td></td><td>Only those ethics committee members who are independent of the clinical trial and the sponsor of the trial should vote /provide opinion in matters related to the study</td></tr>
</table>

Contd...

<table>
<tr><th>Criteria</th><th>ICH-GCP</th><th>Indian GCP</th><th>ICMR Code</th><th>Schedule Y</th></tr>
<tr><td rowspan="2">Non-members with expertise in special areas</td><td rowspan="2">An IRB/IEC may invite nonmembers with expertise in special areas for assistance</td><td colspan="3">If required subject experts could (Schedule Y – may) be invited to offer their views</td></tr>
<tr><td>IRB/IEC may invite for assistance but should not take part in decision making process. However their opinion must be recorded</td><td>For instance, a pediatrician for pediatric conditions, a cardiologist for cardiac disorders etc.</td><td></td></tr>
<tr><td>Representative of patient groups</td><td>Not specified clearly</td><td>Representative of the patient groups or interest groups can be invited during deliberations to offer their viewpoint</td><td colspan="2">Based on the requirement of research area, e.g. HIV AIDS, genetic disorders etc. (ICMR – it is desirable to include a member from specific patient groups in the Committee) (Schedule Y – specific patient groups may also be represented in the EC as far as possible)</td></tr>
<tr><td>Other</td><td></td><td colspan="2">The EC (Indian GCP – at any institution) can have as its members, individuals from other institutions or communities (Indian GCP – If required)</td><td></td></tr>
</table>

Note:

(a) According to Indian GCP and ICMR Code, the **EC composition** may be as follows:

(1) Chairperson (from outside the institute)
(2) 1–2 (ICMR persons from basic medical science area) medical scientists (preferably one pharmacologist)
(3) 1–2 clinicians from various institutes
(4) One legal expert or retired judge
(5) One social scientist/representative of non-governmental voluntary agency
(6) One philosopher/ethicist/theologian
(7) One layperson from the community
(8) Member Secretary (generally belongs to the same institution)

(b) Revised Schedule Y of D&C Act – For review of each protocol, the **Quorum of EC** should be at least 5 members with the following representations:

(1) Basic medical scientists (preferably one pharmacologist)
(2) Clinicians
(3) Legal expert
(4) Social scientist/representative of non-governmental voluntary agency/ philosopher/ethicist/theologian or a similar person
(5) Layperson from the community

DOCUMENTS FOR IRB/IEC SUBMISSION

<table>
<tr><td>Regulatory approval</td><td colspan="2">Indian GCP and ICMR – Relevant regulatory clearances/approvals</td></tr>
<tr><td rowspan="2">Trial procedures and conduct-related documents</td><td colspan="2">Clinical Trial Protocol and Protocol Amendments (if any)</td></tr>
<tr><td colspan="2">CRF (if applicable)</td></tr>
<tr><td rowspan="5">Trial subjects-related documents</td><td>Written Informed Consent Form (ICF) and ICF updates, if any that the investigator proposes for use in the trial</td><td rowspan="2">Indian GCP and ICMR – In both English and vernacular/ local languages</td></tr>
<tr><td>Any other additional written information to be provided to subjects (Indian GCP & ICMR – sample of patient information sheet; PIS)</td></tr>
<tr><td colspan="2">Documents providing information pertaining to amount, methods, and schedule of payments, compensation and expenses available to subjects</td></tr>
<tr><td colspan="2">Subject recruitment procedures e.g. advertisement for subject recruitment (if used/any)</td></tr>
<tr><td colspan="2">Any other documents given approval or favorable opinion (if applicable)</td></tr>
<tr><td rowspan="2">IP-related documents</td><td colspan="2">Investigator's brochure (IB)</td></tr>
<tr><td colspan="2">Any other available safety information</td></tr>
<tr><td rowspan="4">Investigator-related documents</td><td colspan="2">Updated/recent CVs of Principal Investigator, Sub-Investigators and other Consultant Investigators, if any (indicating qualification and experience)</td></tr>
<tr><td colspan="2">Other documents evidencing qualification, experience, training, and license of personnel stated above</td></tr>
<tr><td colspan="2">Investigator's Undertaking Agreement (if required by IRB)</td></tr>
<tr><td colspan="2">Financial Agreement between Sponsor and study site or Investigator (if required by IRB)</td></tr>
<tr><td rowspan="5">Administrative documents (as required by the sponsor)</td><td colspan="2">An official cover letter stating in brief the purpose and summary of trial to be conducted</td></tr>
<tr><td colspan="2">A letter requesting the rapid review of all documents being submitted</td></tr>
<tr><td colspan="2">A letter requesting for interim review of trial conduct at appropriate intervals (as per sponsor's requirements) but not less than once per year</td></tr>
<tr><td colspan="2">List of authorized personnel to be contacted by IRB, with all contact details (representatives from Sponsor, Study site, Pathology lab, CRO, if any)</td></tr>
<tr><td colspan="2">List of documents to be obtained from IRB</td></tr>
<tr><td colspan="3">Any other documents required by IRB/IEC</td></tr>
</table>

Note: Shaded cells in the above table refer to essential documents for a clinical trial to be approved by IRB/IEC as per both ICH-GCP and Indian GCP.

DOCUMENTS TO BE OBTAINED FROM IRB/IEC

<table>
<tr><td colspan="2">Dated, documented approval/favorable opinion of IRB/IEC of the trial for the documents submitted to IRB/IEC for its approval/favorable opinion (the purpose is to document that the trial has been subjected to IRB/IEC review and given approval/favorable opinion and to identify the version number and date of the approved documents)</td></tr>
<tr><td colspan="2">Documents of IRB/IEC composition</td></tr>
<tr><td colspan="2">Documents evidencing the qualifications of IRB members</td></tr>
<tr><td colspan="2">Registration/Accreditation Certificate (stating the authority under which it is established)</td></tr>
<tr><td colspan="2">Statement of independency – Stating that IRB operates independent of institution and/or Investigator (They are not the members of and not being involved in IRB meetings, however they can provide information on any aspect of trial to IRB), IRB may invite members/personnel with expertise in special areas for assistance</td></tr>
<tr><td colspan="2">Criteria for expedited IRB review</td></tr>
<tr><td rowspan="5">Documents by IRB/ IEC Chairperson stating or including (as applicable):</td><td>Statement stating that IRB has written operating procedure and functions accordingly. (e.g. plan for proposed meeting schedule, criteria for evaluation of trial-related documents for review and approval, Plan and frequency of trial review)</td></tr>
<tr><td>Statement stating that IRB maintains written records of
• All its trial related activities
• All trial-related communications
• Minutes of meetings (purpose, discussion held, decisions, members attended/presented, date)</td></tr>
<tr><td>Statement of adherence/compliance with GCP and applicable regulatory authorities</td></tr>
<tr><td>Statement stating the expedited review and providing rapid opinion/ decisions on minor changes/modifications in ongoing previously approved trials according to the criteria provided for expedited review.</td></tr>
<tr><td>Statement stating the maintenance and retention of all Trial-related documents for a Period of at least [Indian GCP – 3; ICH-GCP – 5] years if it is not possible to maintain the same permanently and make them available for regulatory inspection and will notify sponsor/institution/investigator before the displacement/destruction of trial documents)</td></tr>
</table>

Note: Shaded cells in the above table refer to essential documents for a clinical trial to be obtained from IRB/IEC as per both ICH-GCP and Indian GCP.

ESSENTIAL DOCUMENTS FOR THE CONDUCT OF A CLINICAL TRIAL

Note:

1. The term "site" is equivalent to 'investigator/institution'.
2. Essential documents to be retained in the files of both Investigator (site) and Sponsor are mainly based on ICH-GCP; however requirements of Indian GCP have also been described and following denotations have been used.
   - Symbol "**X**" means 'required by both ICH and Indian GCP'
   - Symbol "**RIG**" means "required by Indian GCP'
   - Symbol "**NA**" means 'not required by both ICH and Indian GCP'
   - Symbol "**NRIG**" means 'not required by Indian GCP'
3. Essential documents to be retained in the files of CRO and IRB/IEC are described by only Indian GCP.
   - Symbols both "X" and "RIG" mean 'required by Indian GCP'
   - Symbol "NRIG" means 'not required by Indian GCP'

Before the Clinical Phase of the Trial Commences

<table>
<tr><th colspan="2" rowspan="3">Title of the Document</th><th colspan="4">Required to be Located in Files of</th><th rowspan="3">Purpose</th></tr>
<tr><th colspan="2">Described by both ICH and Indian GCP</th><th colspan="2">Described by Indian GCP</th></tr>
<tr><th>Site</th><th>Sponsor</th><th>CRO</th><th>IRB/IEC</th></tr>
<tr><td colspan="2">Investigator's brochure</td><td>X</td><td>X</td><td>X</td><td>X</td><td>To document that relevant and current scientific information about the investigational product has been provided to the investigator</td></tr>
<tr><td colspan="2">Signed Protocol and Amendments, if any</td><td>X</td><td>X</td><td>X</td><td>X</td><td>To document investigator and sponsor agreement to the protocol/amendments</td></tr>
<tr><td colspan="2">Sample case report form (CRF)</td><td>X</td><td>X</td><td>X</td><td>X</td><td>To document investigator and sponsor agreement to the CRF</td></tr>
<tr><td rowspan="2">Infor-mation given to trial sub-jects</td><td>Informed consent form (including all applicable translations)</td><td>X</td><td>X</td><td>X</td><td>X</td><td>To document the informed consent</td></tr>
<tr><td>Any other written infor-mation</td><td>X</td><td>X</td><td>X</td><td>X</td><td>To document that subjects will be given appropriate written information (content and word-ing) to support their ability to give fully informed consent</td></tr>
<tr><td></td><td>Advertise-ment for subject recruitment (if used)</td><td>X</td><td>RIG</td><td>X</td><td>X</td><td>To document that recruitment measures are appropriate and not coercive</td></tr>
</table>

Contd...

<table>
<tr><th colspan="2" rowspan="3">Title of the Document</th><th colspan="4">Required to be Located in Files of</th><th rowspan="3">Purpose</th></tr>
<tr><th colspan="2">Described by both ICH and Indian GCP</th><th colspan="2">Described by Indian GCP</th></tr>
<tr><th>Site</th><th>Sponsor</th><th>CRO</th><th>IRB/IEC</th></tr>
<tr><td colspan="2">Financial aspects of the trial</td><td>X</td><td>X</td><td>X</td><td>X</td><td>To document the financial agreement between the investigator/institution and the sponsor for the trial</td></tr>
<tr><td colspan="2">Insurance statement (where required)</td><td>X</td><td>X</td><td>X</td><td>X</td><td>To document that compensation to subjects for trial-related injury will be available</td></tr>
<tr><td rowspan="4">Signed agreement between involved parties</td><td>Investigator/ institution and sponsor</td><td>X (NRIG)</td><td>X (NRIG)</td><td>NRIG</td><td>NRIG</td><td rowspan="4">To document agreements</td></tr>
<tr><td>Investigator/ institution and CRO</td><td>X (NRIG)</td><td>X (NRIG)</td><td>NRIG</td><td>NRIG</td></tr>
<tr><td>Sponsor and CRO</td><td>NA</td><td>X (where required) (NRIG)</td><td>NRIG</td><td>NRIG</td></tr>
<tr><td>Investigator/ institution and authorities (where required)</td><td>X (NRIG)</td><td>X (NRIG)</td><td>NRIG</td><td>NRIG</td></tr>
<tr><td rowspan="7">Dated documented approval/ favourable opinion of IRB/IEC of the</td><td>Protocol and any amendments</td><td rowspan="7">X</td><td rowspan="7">X</td><td rowspan="7">X</td><td rowspan="7">X</td><td rowspan="7">To document that the trial has been subject to IRB/IEC review and given approval/favourable opinion. To identify the version number and date of the documents</td></tr>
<tr><td>CRF (if applicable)</td></tr>
<tr><td>Informed consent forms</td></tr>
<tr><td>Any other written information to be provided to the subjects</td></tr>
<tr><td>Advertisement for subject recruitment (if used)</td></tr>
<tr><td>Subject compensation (if any)</td></tr>
<tr><td>Any other documents given approval/ favourable opinion</td></tr>
</table>

Contd...

Title of the Document	Required to be Located in Files of				Purpose
	Described by both ICH and Indian GCP		Described by Indian GCP		
	Site	Sponsor	CRO	IRB/IEC	
IRB/IEC composition	X	X (where required as per ICH-GCP)	X	X	To document that the IRB/IEC is constituted in agreement with GCP
Regulatory authorities authorization/ approval/notification of protocol (where required)	X (where required)	X (where required)	X	X	To document appropriate authorisation/approval/notification by the regulatory authorities has been prior to initiation of the trial in compliance with the applicable regulatory requirements
Curriculum vitae and/ or other relevant documents evidencing qualifications of investigators and (Indian GCP – co-investigator) sub-investigators	X	X	X	X	To document qualifications and eligibility to conduct trial and/ or provide medical supervision of subjects
Normal value(s)/ range(s) for medical/ laboratory/technical procedures and/or tests included in the Protocol	X	X	X	NRIG	To document normal values and/or ranges of the tests
Medical/laboratory/ technical procedures / tests • certification or • accreditation or • established quality control and/or external quality assessment or • other validation (where required) (Indian GCP – these documents are to be filed in 'during the trial' section of essential documents)	X (where required) (NRIG)	X (NRIG)	X (NRIG)	X (NRIG)	To document competence of facility to perform required tests and support reliability of results
Sample of labels attached to investigational product containers	RIG	X	X	NRIG	To document compliance with applicable labelling regulations and appropriateness of instructions provided to the subjects
Instructions for handling of investigational product(s) and trial-related materials and supplies (if not included in protocol or investigator's brochure)	X	X	X	NRIG	To document instructions needed to ensure proper storage, packaging, dispensing and disposition of IP(s) and trial-related materials

Contd...

<table>
<tr><th colspan="2" rowspan="3">Title of the Document</th><th colspan="4">Required to be Located in Files of</th><th rowspan="3">Purpose</th></tr>
<tr><th colspan="2">Described by both ICH and Indian GCP</th><th colspan="2">Described by Indian GCP</th></tr>
<tr><th>Site</th><th>Sponsor</th><th>CRO</th><th>IRB/IEC</th></tr>
<tr><td colspan="2">Shipping records for investigational product(s) and trial-related material</td><td>X</td><td>X</td><td>X</td><td>NRIG</td><td>To document shipment dates, batch numbers and method of shipment of investigational product(s) and trial-related materials. Allows tracking of product batch, review of shipping conditions, and accountability</td></tr>
<tr><td colspan="2">Certificate(s) of analysis of investigational product(s) shipped</td><td>NA</td><td>X</td><td>X</td><td>NRIG</td><td>To document identity, purity, and strength of investigational product(s) to be used in the trial</td></tr>
<tr><td colspan="2">Decoding procedures for blinded trials</td><td>X</td><td>X (third party if applicable) (RIG)</td><td>X</td><td>NRIG</td><td>To document how, in case of an emergency, identity of blinded investigational product can be revealed without breaking the blind for the remaining subjects' treatment</td></tr>
<tr><td colspan="2">Master randomization list</td><td>NA</td><td>X (third party if applicable) (RIG)</td><td>X</td><td>NRIG</td><td>To document method for randomisation of trial population</td></tr>
<tr><td rowspan="2">These both reports may be combined with each other</td><td>Pre-trial monitoring report</td><td>NA</td><td>X</td><td>X</td><td>NRIG</td><td>To document that the site is suitable for the trial (may be combined with trial initiation monitoring report)</td></tr>
<tr><td>Trial initiation monitoring report</td><td>X</td><td>X</td><td>X</td><td>NRIG</td><td>To document that trial procedures were reviewed with the investigator and the investigator's trial staff (may be combined with pre-trial monitoring reports)</td></tr>
</table>

During the Clinical Conduct of the Trial

<table>
<tr><th rowspan="3">Title of the Document</th><th colspan="4">Required to be Located in Files of</th><th rowspan="3">Purpose</th></tr>
<tr><th colspan="2">Described by both ICH and Indian GCP</th><th colspan="2">Described by Indian GCP</th></tr>
<tr><th>Site</th><th>Sponsor</th><th>CRO</th><th>IRB/IEC</th></tr>
<tr><td>Investigator's brochure updates</td><td>X</td><td>X</td><td>X</td><td>X</td><td>To document that investigator is informed in a timely manner of relevant information as it becomes available</td></tr>
</table>

Contd...

<table>
<tr><th colspan="3" rowspan="3">Title of the Document</th><th colspan="4">Required to be Located in Files of</th><th rowspan="3">Purpose</th></tr>
<tr><th colspan="2">Described by both ICH and Indian GCP</th><th colspan="2">Described by Indian GCP</th></tr>
<tr><th>Site</th><th>Sponsor</th><th>CRO</th><th>IRB/IEC</th></tr>
<tr><td rowspan="5">Any revisions to</td><td colspan="2">Protocol/amendments</td><td>X</td><td>X</td><td>X</td><td>X</td><td rowspan="5">To document revisions of these trial related documents that take effect during trial</td></tr>
<tr><td colspan="2">Case report form (CRF)</td><td>X</td><td>X</td><td>X</td><td>X</td></tr>
<tr><td colspan="2">Informed consent form</td><td>X</td><td>X</td><td>X</td><td>X</td></tr>
<tr><td colspan="2">Any other written information provided to subjects</td><td>X</td><td>X</td><td>X</td><td>X</td></tr>
<tr><td colspan="2">Advertisements for subject recruitment (if used)</td><td>X</td><td>X</td><td>X</td><td>X</td></tr>
<tr><td rowspan="6">Dated, Documented Approval/ Favorable Opinion of IRB/IEC of the</td><td colspan="2">Protocol amendments</td><td>X</td><td>X</td><td>X</td><td>X</td><td rowspan="6">To document that the amendments and/or revisions have been subject to IRB/IEC review and were given approval/favourable opinion. To identify the version number and date of the documents</td></tr>
<tr><td rowspan="3">Revisions of</td><td>Informed consent form</td><td>X</td><td>X</td><td>X</td><td>X</td></tr>
<tr><td>Any other written information to be provided to the subjects</td><td>X</td><td>X</td><td>X</td><td>X</td></tr>
<tr><td>Advertisements for subject recruitment (if used)</td><td>X</td><td>X</td><td>X</td><td>X</td></tr>
<tr><td colspan="2">Any other documents given approval/favorable opinion</td><td>X</td><td>X</td><td>X</td><td>X</td></tr>
<tr><td colspan="2">Continuing review of trial (where required)</td><td>X</td><td>X</td><td>X</td><td>X</td></tr>
<tr><td colspan="3">Regulatory authorities authorizations/approvals/notifications where required for Protocol amendments and other regulatory documents</td><td>X (where required) (RIG)</td><td>X</td><td>X</td><td>X</td><td>To document compliance with applicable regulatory requirements</td></tr>
</table>

Contd...

Title of the Document	Required to be Located in Files of				Purpose
	Described by both ICH and Indian GCP		Described by Indian GCP		
	Site	Sponsor	CRO	IRB/IEC	
Curriculum vitae for new investigators and/or sub-investigators	X	X	X	X	To document qualifications and eligibility to conduct trial and/or provide medical supervision of subjects
Updates to normal values/ranges for medical/laboratory/technical procedures/tests included in the Protocol	X	X	X	NRIG	To document normal values and ranges that are revised during the trial in addition to document normal values and/or ranges of the tests
Updates of medical/laboratory/technical procedures/tests • certification or • accreditation or • established quality control and/or external quality assessment or • other validation (where required) (Indian GCP – the before trial documents of these documents are to be filed here)	X (where required) (RIG)	X	X	NRIG	To document that tests remain adequate throughout the trial period in addition to document competence of facility to perform required tests and support reliability of results
Documentation of investigational products and trial-related materials shipment	X	X	X	NRIG	To document shipment dates, batch numbers and method of shipment of investigational products and trial-related materials. Allows tracking of product batch, review of shipping conditions, and accountability
Certificates of analysis for new batches of investigational products	NA	X	X	NRIG	To document identity, purity, and strength of investigational products to be used in the trial
Monitoring visit reports	NA	X	X	NRIG	To document site visits by, and findings of, the monitor
Relevant communications other than site visits • letters • meeting notes • notes of telephone calls	X	X (NRIG)	X	NRIG	To document any agreements or significant discussions regarding trial administration, protocol violations, trial conduct, adverse event (AE) reporting

Contd...

Title of the Document	Required to be Located in Files of				Purpose
	Described by both ICH and Indian GCP		Described by Indian GCP		
	Site	Sponsor	CRO	IRB/IEC	
Signed iInformed consent forms	X (RIG – Original)	(RIG-Copy)	(RIG-Copy)	NRIG	To document that consent is obtained in accordance with GCP and protocol and dated prior to participation of each subject in trial. Also to document direct access permission. Also to document the purposes as described in 'Information given to subjects' in the section of before trial
Source documents	X (RIG – Original)	(RIG-Copy)	(RIG-Copy)	NRIG	To document the existence of the subject and substantiate integrity of trial data collected. To include original documents related to the trial, to medical treatment, and history of subject
Signed, dated and completed case report forms (CRF)	X (Copy)	X (Original) (RIG-Copy)	X (Copy)	NRIG	To document that the investigator or authorised member of the investigator's staff confirms the observations recorded
Documentation of CRF corrections	X (Copy) (RIG-Original)	X (Original) (RIG-Copy)	X (Copy)	NRIG	To document all changes/additions or corrections made to CRF after initial data were recorded
Notification by originating investigator to sponsor of serious adverse events and related reports	X	X	X	X	Notification by originating investigator to sponsor of serious adverse events and related reports in accordance with the regulatory requirements of safety reporting

Contd...

Title of the Document	Required to be Located in Files of				Purpose
	Described by both ICH and Indian GCP		Described by Indian GCP		
	Site	Sponsor	CRO	IRB/IEC	
Notification by sponsor and/or Investigator, where applicable, to regulatory authorities and IRBs/IECs of unexpected serious adverse drug reactions and of other safety information	X (where re-quired) (RIG)	X	X	X	Notification by sponsor and/or investigator, where applicable, to regulatory authorities and IRBs/IECs of unexpected serious adverse drug reactions and of other safety information in accordance with regulatory requirements for safety reporting
Notification by sponsor to investigators of safety information	X	X	X	X	Notification by sponsor to investigators of safety information in accordance with requirements of safety reporting
Interim or annual reports to IRB/IEC and authorities	X	X (where required) (RIG)	X	X	Interim or annual reports provided to IRB/IEC in accordance with requirements of reporting progress reports and to authority(ies) in accordance with requirements for safety reporting
Subject screening log	X	X (where required)	X (where re-quired)	NRIG	To document identification of subjects who entered pre-trial screening
Subject identification code list	X	RIG	X	NRIG	To document that investigator/institution keeps a confidential list of names of all subjects allocated to trial numbers on enrolling in the trial. Allows investigator/institution to reveal identity of any subject
Subject enrollment log	X	RIG	X	NRIG	To document chronological enrolment of subjects by trial number
Investigational products accountability at the site	X	X	X	NRIG	To document that investigational products have been used according to the protocol

Contd...

Title of the Document	Required to be Located in Files of				Purpose
	Described by both ICH and Indian GCP		Described by Indian GCP		
	Site	Sponsor	CRO	IRB/IEC	
Signature sheet	X	X	X	NRIG	To document signatures and initials of all persons authorised to make entries and/or corrections on CRFs
Record of retained body fluids/ tissue samples (if any)	X	X	X	NRIG	To document location and identification of retained samples if assays need to be repeated

After Completion or Termination of the Trial

Title of the Document	Required to be Located in Files of				Purpose
	Described by both ICH and Indian GCP		Described by Indian GCP		
	Site	Sponsor	CRO	IRB/ IEC	
Investigational products accountability at site	X	X	X	NRIG	To document that the investigational products have been used according to the protocol. To documents the final accounting of investigational products received at the site, dispensed to subjects, returned by the subjects, and returned to sponsor
Documentation of investigational product destruction	X (if destroyed at site)	X	X	NRIG	To document destruction of unused investigational products by sponsor or at site
Completed subject identification code list	X	RIG	X	NRIG	To permit identification of all subjects enrolled in the trial in case follow-up is required. List should be kept in a confidential manner and for agreed upon time
Audit certificate (if available)	NA	X	X	NRIG	To document that audit was performed

Contd...

Title of the Document	Required to be Located in Files of				Purpose
	Described by both ICH and Indian GCP		Described by Indian GCP		
	Site	Spon-sor	CRO	IRB/IEC	
Final trial close-out monitoring report	NA	X	X	NRIG	To document that all activities required for trial close-out are completed, and copies of essential documents are held in the appropriate files
Treatment allocation and decoding documentation	NA	X	X	NRIG	Returned to sponsor to document any decoding that may have occurred
Final report by investigator to IRB/IEC where required, and where applicable, to the regulatory Authorities	X	RIG	X	X	To document completion of the trial
Clinical study report	X (if applicable) (RIG)	X	X	X	To document results and interpretation of trial

Chapter 3

Clinical Trial Framework

A clinical trial framework describes the pathway of a clinical trial from the planning phase up to the completion of the study in a logical and sequential manner. The purpose of this clinical trial framework is to enhance the understanding of GCP and to describe how the various trial activities are interlinked with each other. This framework has been presented in the form of flowcharts. These flowcharts may not necessarily cover all the activities, but can be used for developing a framework based on the specific needs of the study, sponsor and regulations.

This framework is primarily based on ICH-GCP guideline. However, some flowcharts are based on Indian GCP (e.g. prerequisites for the study, IRB decision-making process, and selection of children, pregnant and nursing women, etc.). Some flowcharts (e.g., clinical project assessment, study design, selection of CRO, screening and trial procedure initiation, etc.) are not part of GCP, but are provided to maintain the flow of clinical trial pathway. It is recommended that this clinical trial framework be read in relation with the GCP for a better understanding.

FLOWCHART 1 CLINICAL PROJECT ASSESSMENT

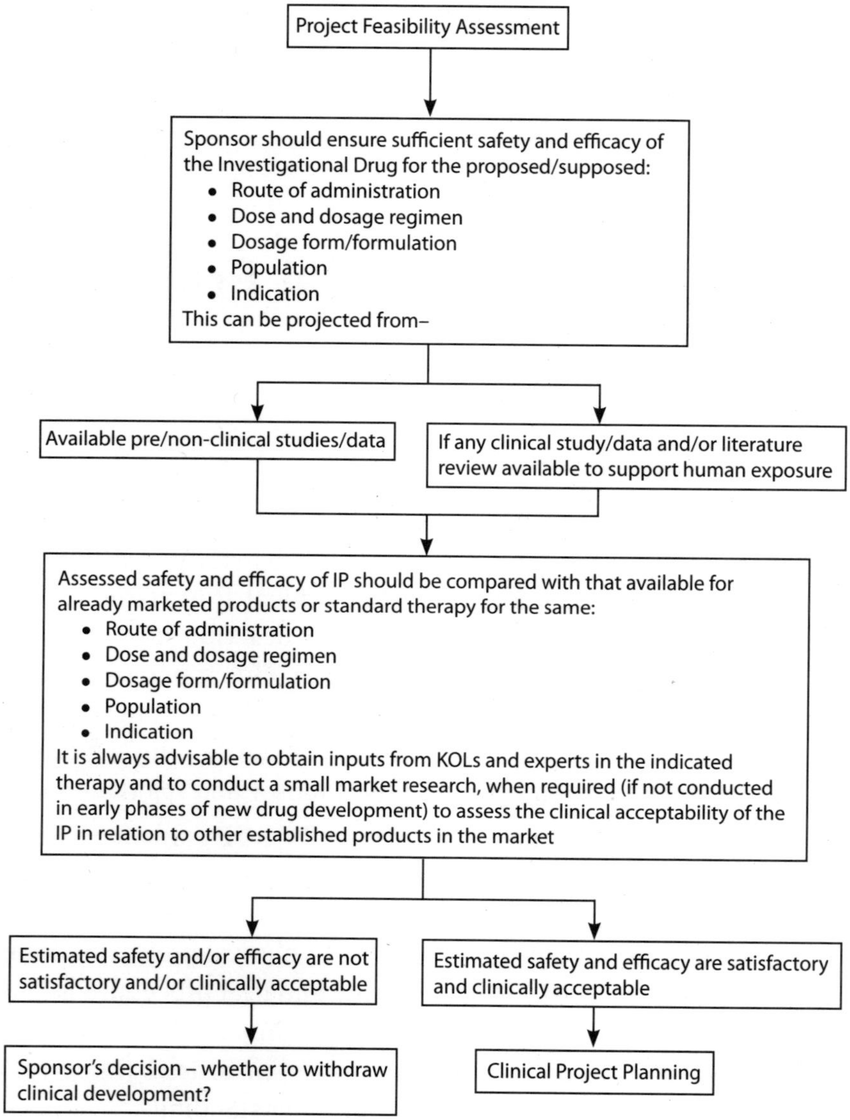

FLOWCHART 2 CLINICAL PROJECT PLANNING

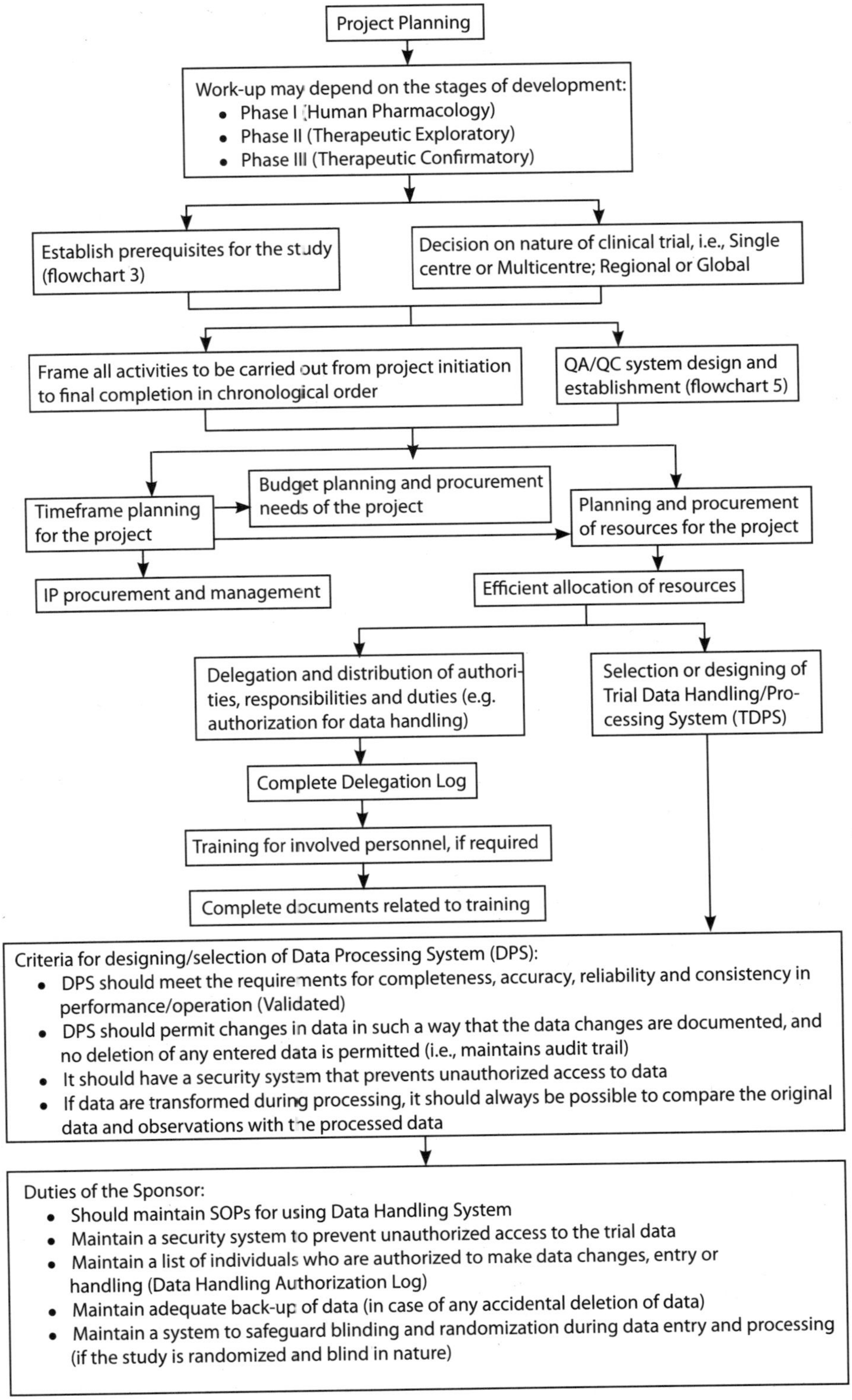

FLOWCHART 3 PREREQUISITES FOR THE STUDY

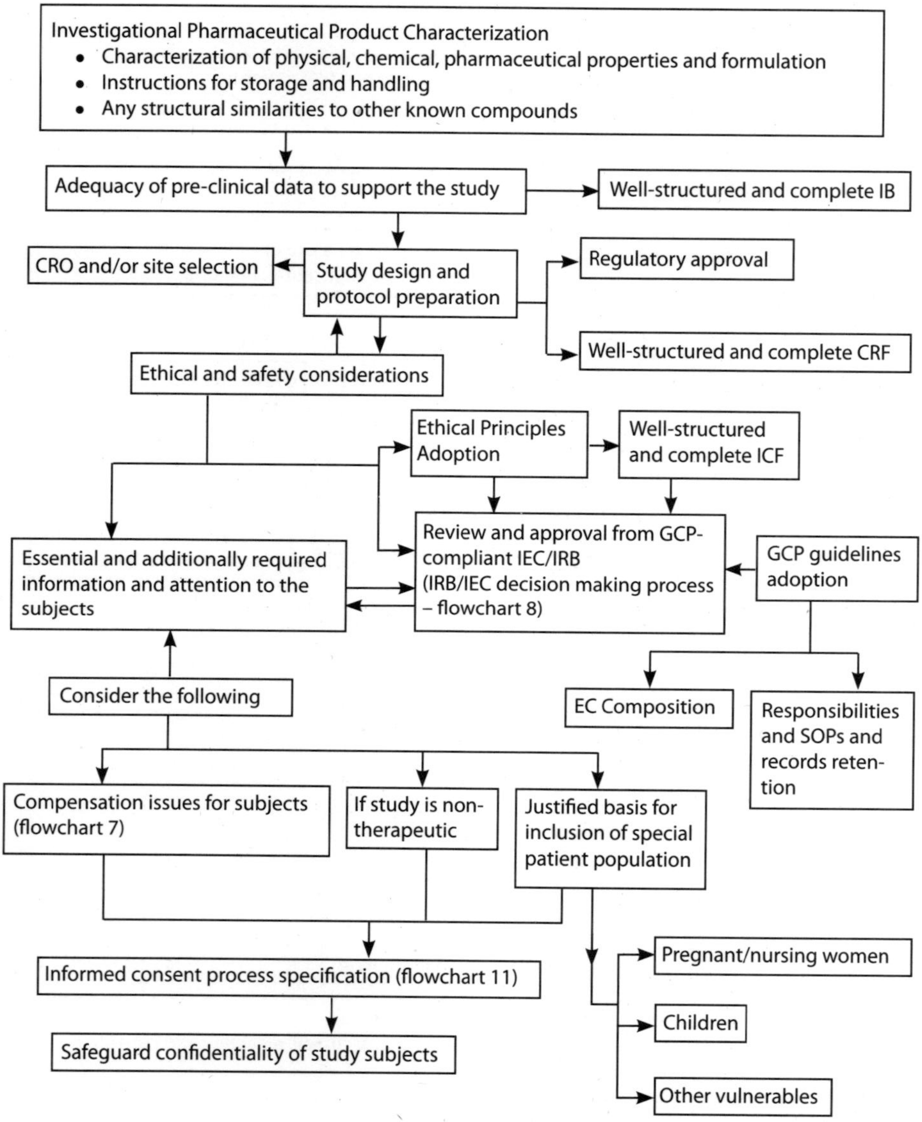

FLOWCHART 4 STUDY DESIGN

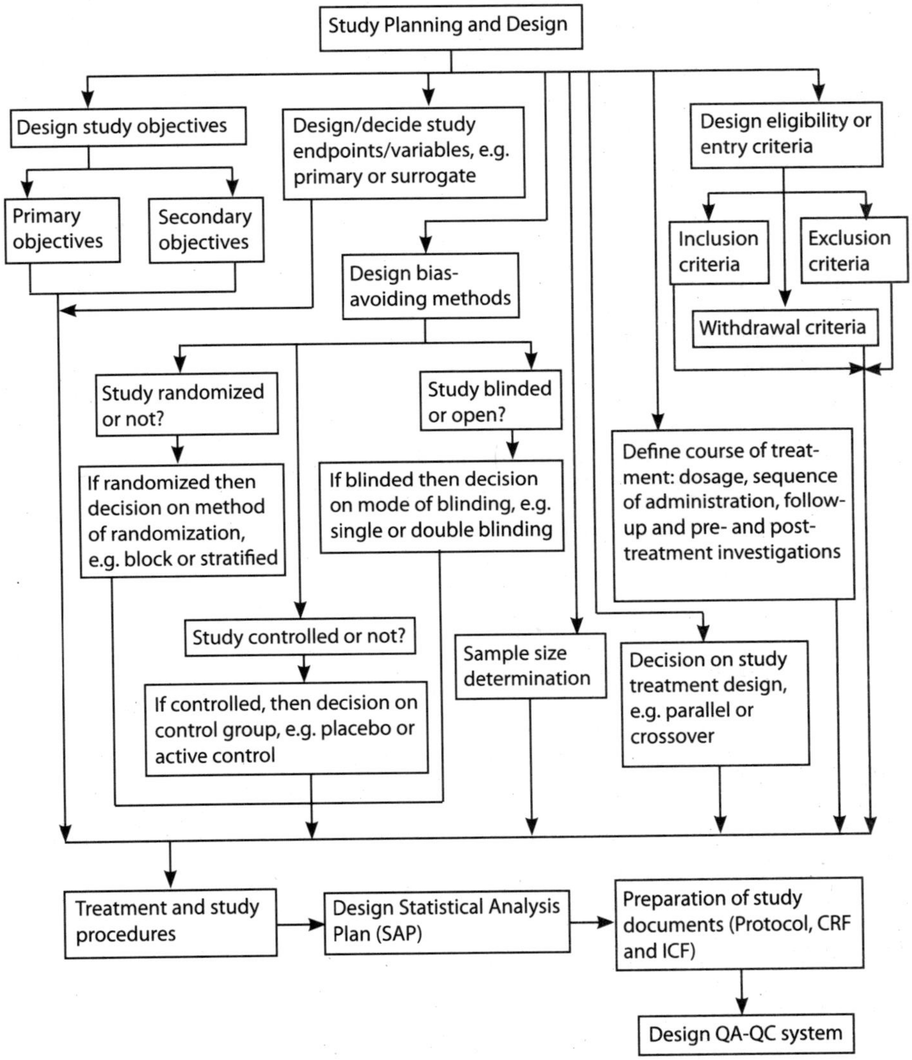

FLOWCHART 5 CLINICAL TRIAL QA-QC SYSTEM

Overall quality of a clinical trial depends on:

1. Quality conduct of trial procedures
2. Quality of
   - data generation
   - data recording
   - data reporting
   - data handling
   - data archival

↓

Objectives of ensuring quality of clinical trials are–

- To maintain compliance of treatment/trial procedures with GCP, Protocols, ARRs
- To assure all captured data are reliable, valid and processed accurately

The quality of trial procedures and data is:

↓

Controlled during the trial period by | Assured after completion of trial by

↓

- Establishment,
- Implementation and
- Control and updating

of quality assurance and quality control system with written SOPs

↓

SOPs for site-related procedures | SOPs for sponsor-related procedures (including monitoring and audit plans)

↓

Before trial procedures | During trial procedures | After trial procedures

↓

Designing and/or deciding the TOC or TMF to prepare checklist of essential documents to be retained in regulatory documents binder of both sponsor and investigator

Designing the formats of trial-related secondary documents for documenting all the activities of trial conduct (this can be done as attached forms, logs with SOPs)

Note: Usually most sponsor companies and CROs have a well-developed quality system, which can be used for all clinical studies by incorporating study-specific requirements into it.

FLOWCHART 6 MANAGEMENT OF IP AND IP-RELATED DOCUMENTS

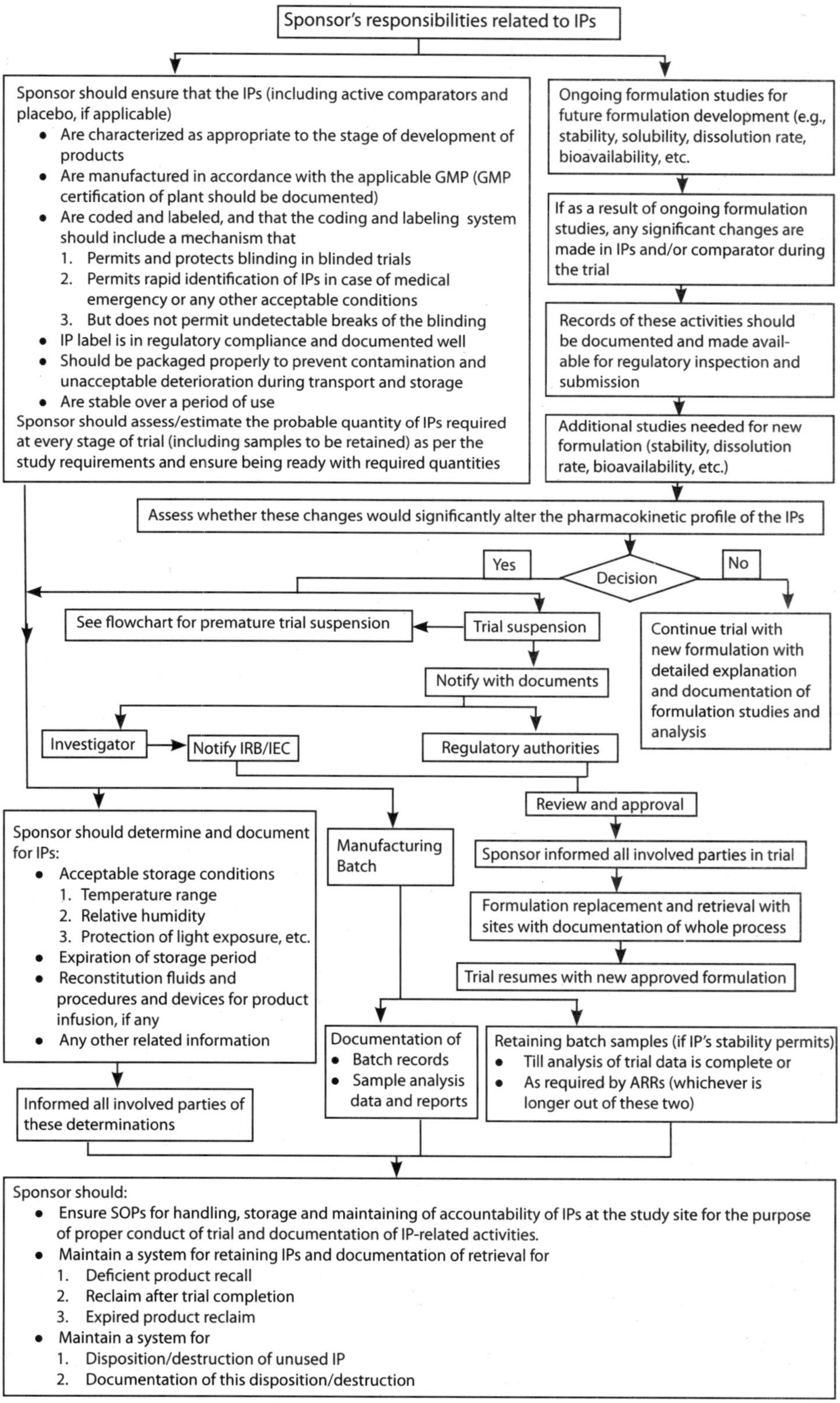

FLOWCHART 7 COMPENSATION FOR SUBJECT'S PARTICIPATION

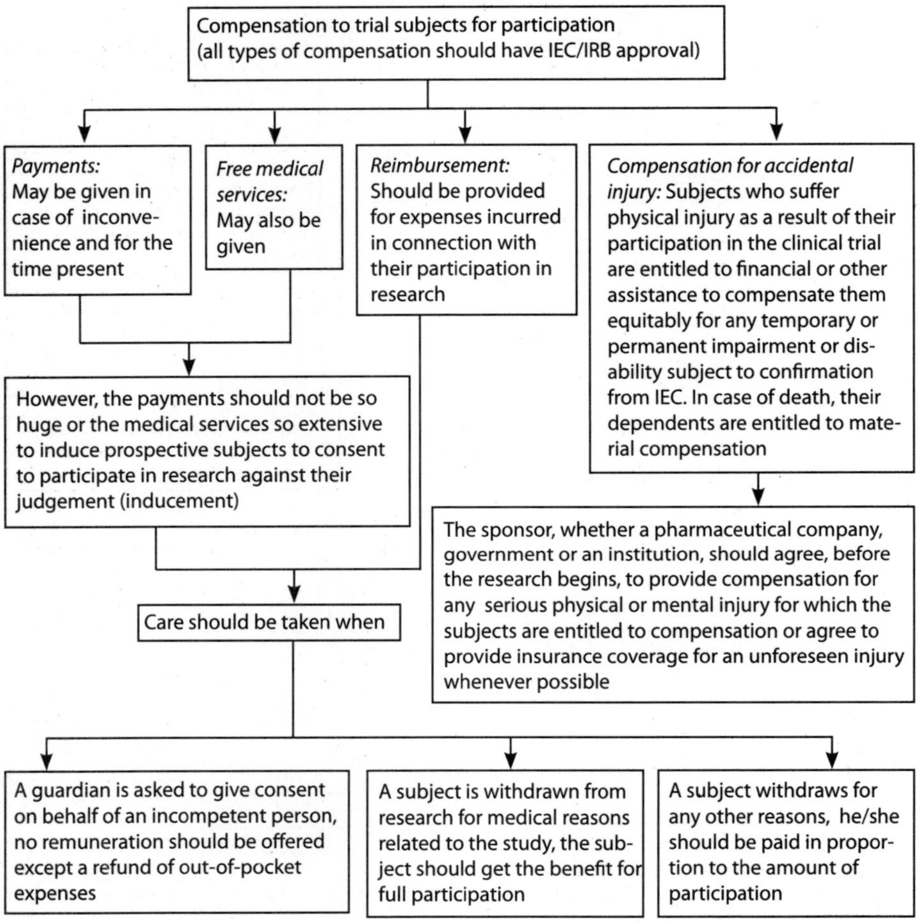

FLOWCHART 8 IRB/IEC DECISION-MAKING PROCESS

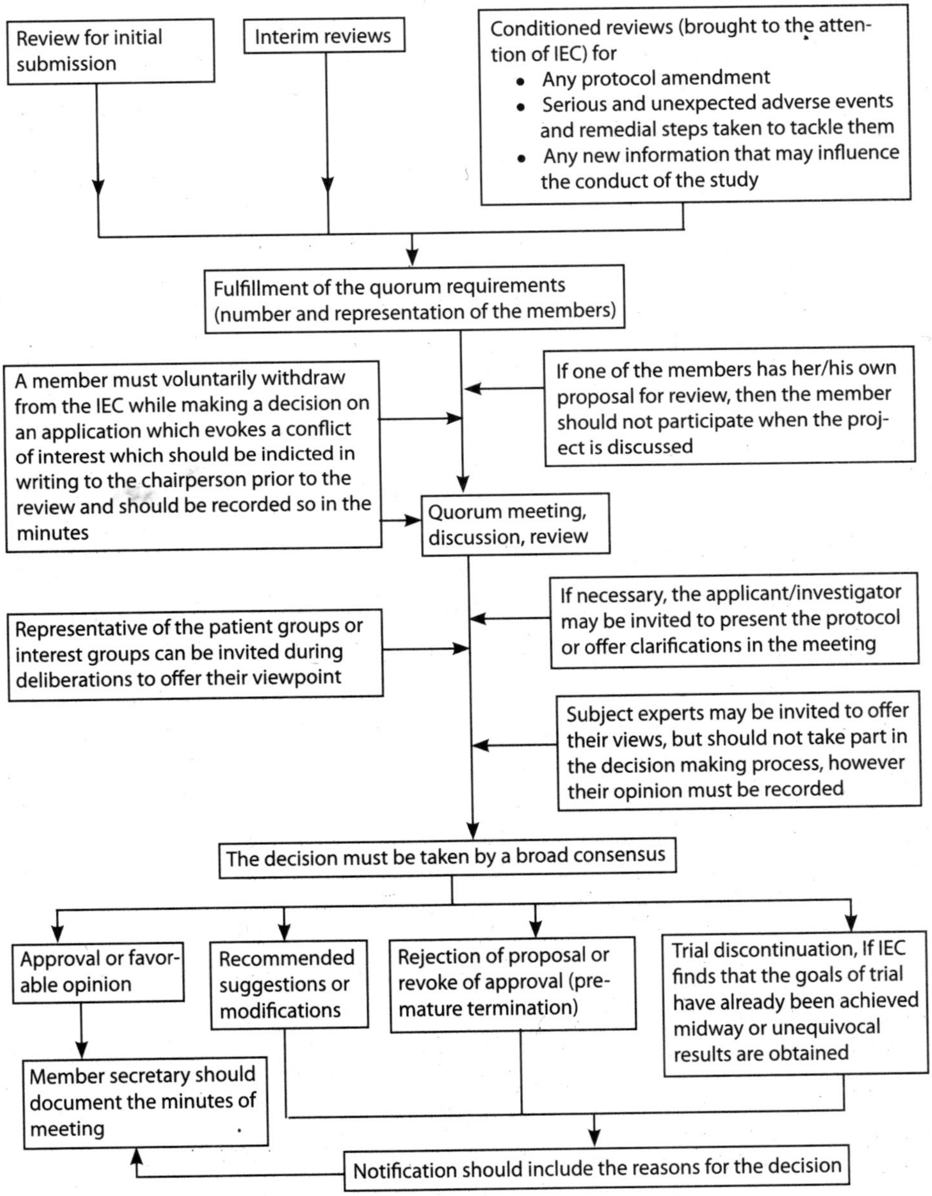

FLOWCHART 9 SELECTION OF CONTRACT RESEARCH ORGANIZATION (CRO)

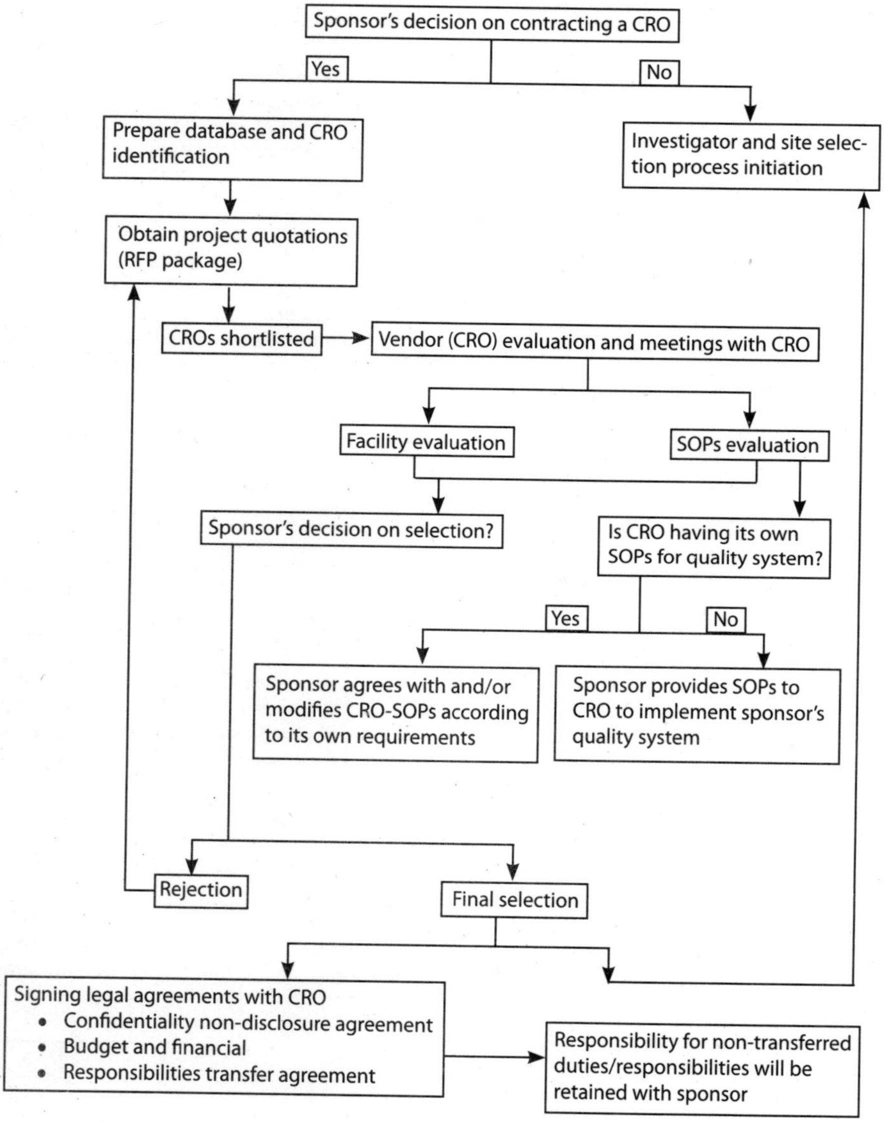

FLOWCHART 10 INVESTIGATOR AND SITE SELECTION

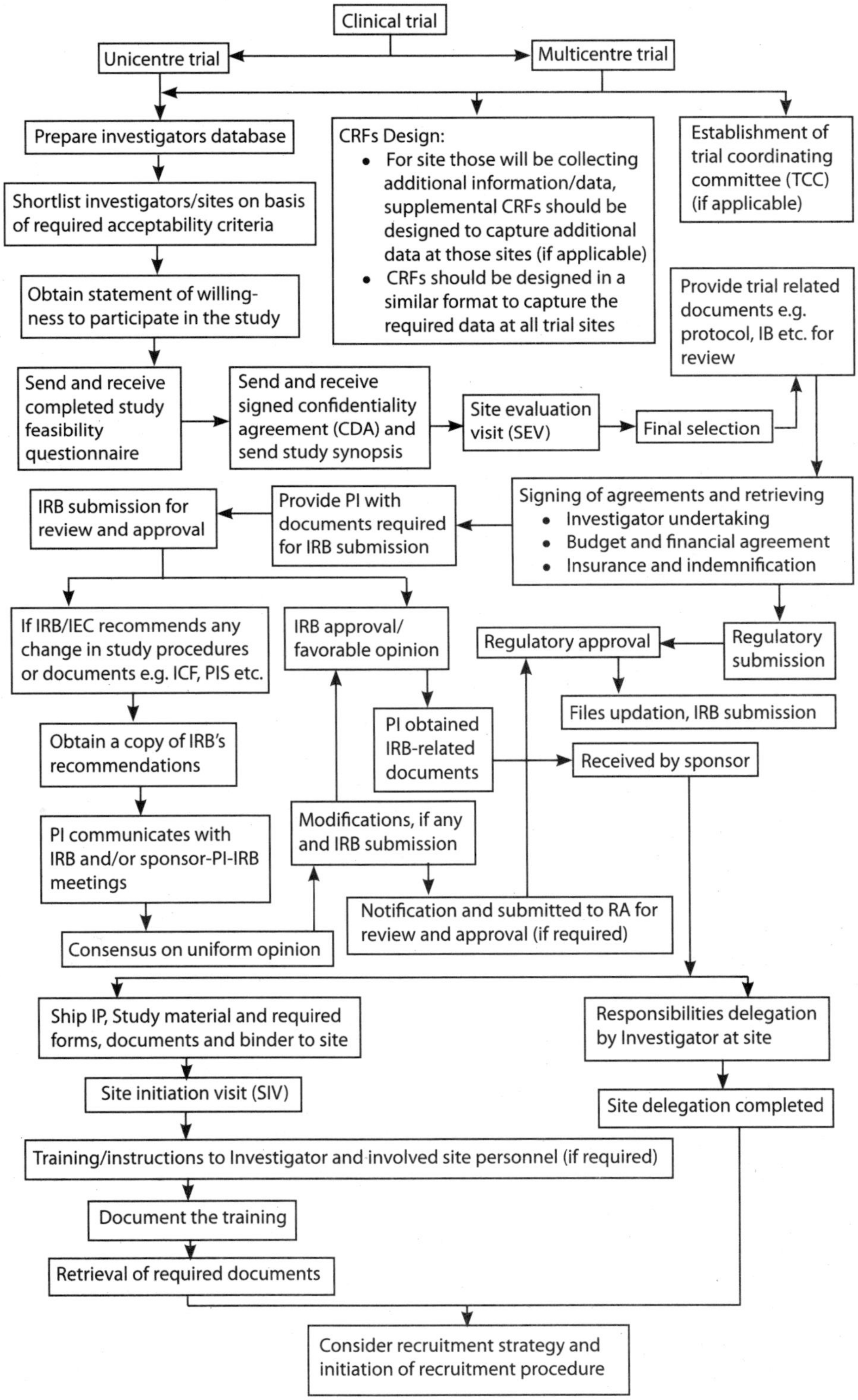

FLOWCHART 11 SUBJECT RECRUITMENT PROCEDURE

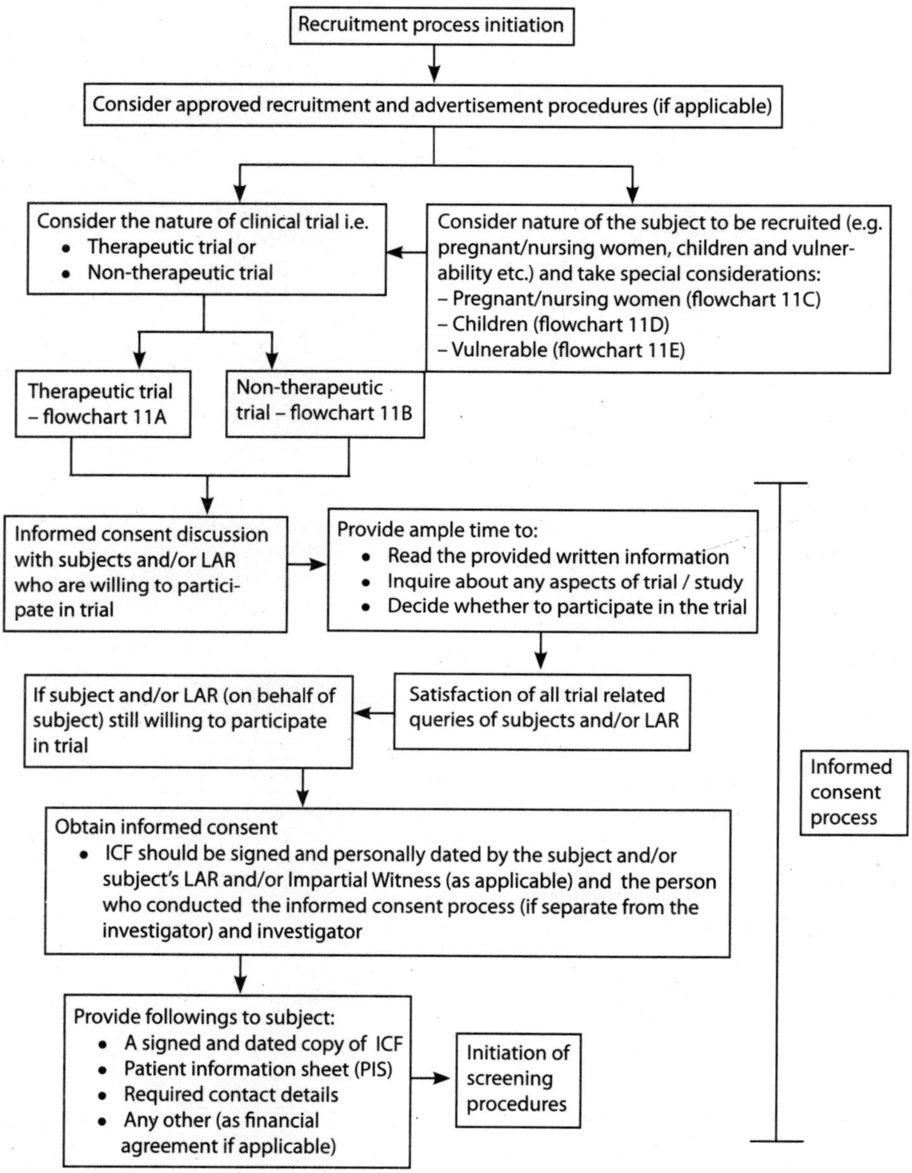

Note: During informed consent discussion, the subject and/or LAR should be fully informed of all pertinent aspects of the trial, including any written information available and approval/favorable opinion given by the IRB/IEC.

FLOWCHART 11A THERAPEUTIC TRIAL

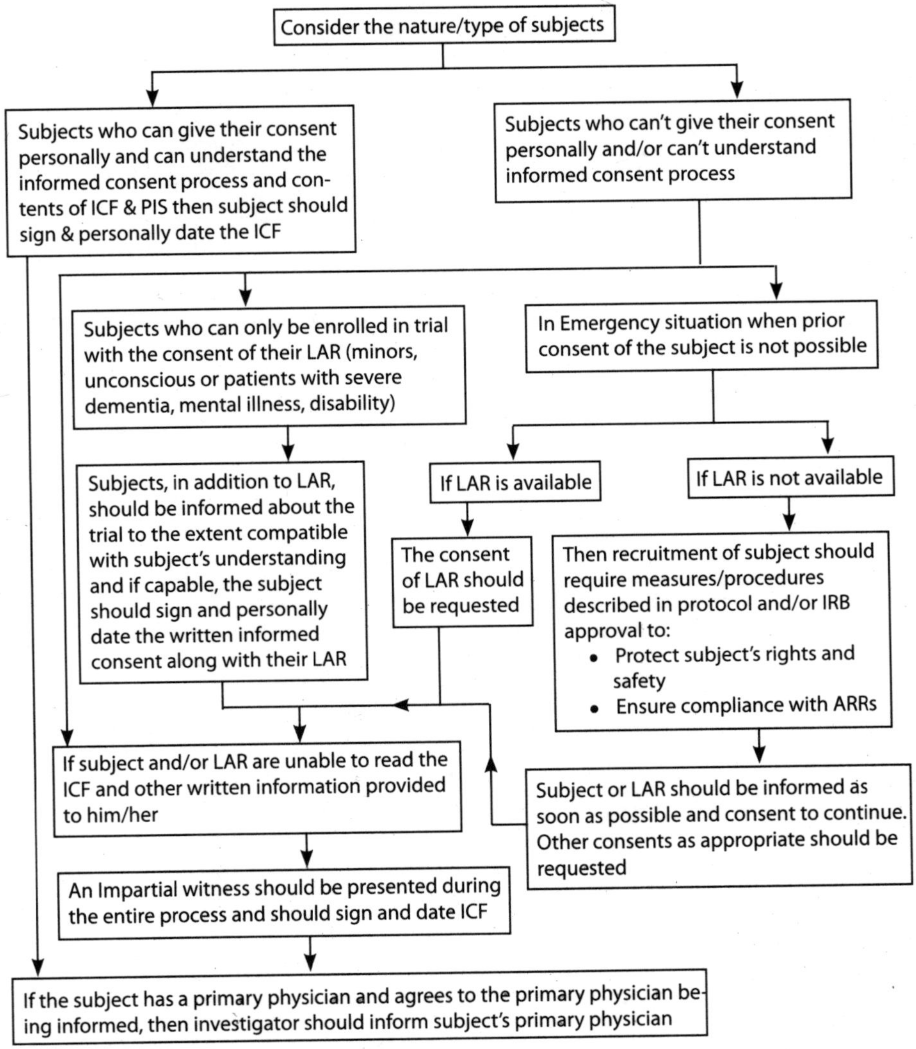

Note: For illiterate subjects and/or LAR, their thumb impression should be taken along with sign and dated by impartial witness.

As a general rule in Indian GCP, a signed form as an evidence of informed consent (written informed consent) preferably witnessed by a person not related to the trial should be obtained from each prospective subject.

FLOWCHART 11B NON-THERAPEUTIC TRIAL

A trial in which there is no anticipated direct clinical benefits to subject

Normal conditions:
Should only be conducted in subjects who personally can give consent and sign and date the ICF personally

Exempted/special/exceptional conditions:
May be conducted in subjects with consent of a LAR if following conditions are fulfilled:

- The objectives of the trial cannot be met by means of a trial in subjects who can give informed consent personally
- The foreseeable risks to the subjects are low
- The negative impact on the subject's wellbeing is minimized and low
- The trial is not prohibited by law
- The approval/favorable opinion of the IRB/IEC is expressly sought on the inclusion of such subjects, and the written approval/favorable opinion covers this aspect

- Such trials unless an exception is justified, should be conducted in patients having a disease or condition for which the IP is intended
- Subjects in these trials should be particularly closely monitored and should be withdrawn if they appear to be unduly distressed

See the flowchart for therapeutic trial

FLOWCHART 11C PREGNANT OR NURSING WOMEN AS RESEARCH SUBJECT

Pregnant or nursing women should in no circumstances be the subject of any research unless the research fulfils both of the following conditions

The research carries no more than minimal risk to the foetus or nursing infant

The object of the research is to obtain new knowledge about the foetus, pregnancy and lactation, to protect or advance the health of pregnant or nursing women or foetuses or nursing infants, and for which women who are not pregnant or nursing would not be suitable subject, e.g.

- To test the efficacy and safety of a drug for reducing perinatal transmission of HIV infection from mother to child
- Trials for detecting foetal abnormalities
- Research for conditions associated with or aggravated by pregnancy

Nursing women:
Women should not be encouraged to discontinue nursing for the sake of participation in research and in case she decides to do so, harm of cessation of breast feeding to the nursing child should be properly assessed except in those studies where breast feeding is harmful to the infant.

Pregnant women

Research related to termination of pregnancy:
Pregnant women who desire to undergo Medical Termination of Pregnancy (MTP) could be made subjects for such research as per Medical Termination of Pregnancy Act, GOI, 1971

Research related to pre-natal diagnostic techniques:
In Pregnant women such research should be limited to detect the foetal abnormalities or genetic disorders as per the Prenatal Diagnostic Techniques (Regulation and Prevention of Misuse) Act, GOI, 1994 and not for sex determination of the foetus

FLOWCHART 11D CHILDREN AS RESEARCH SUBJECT

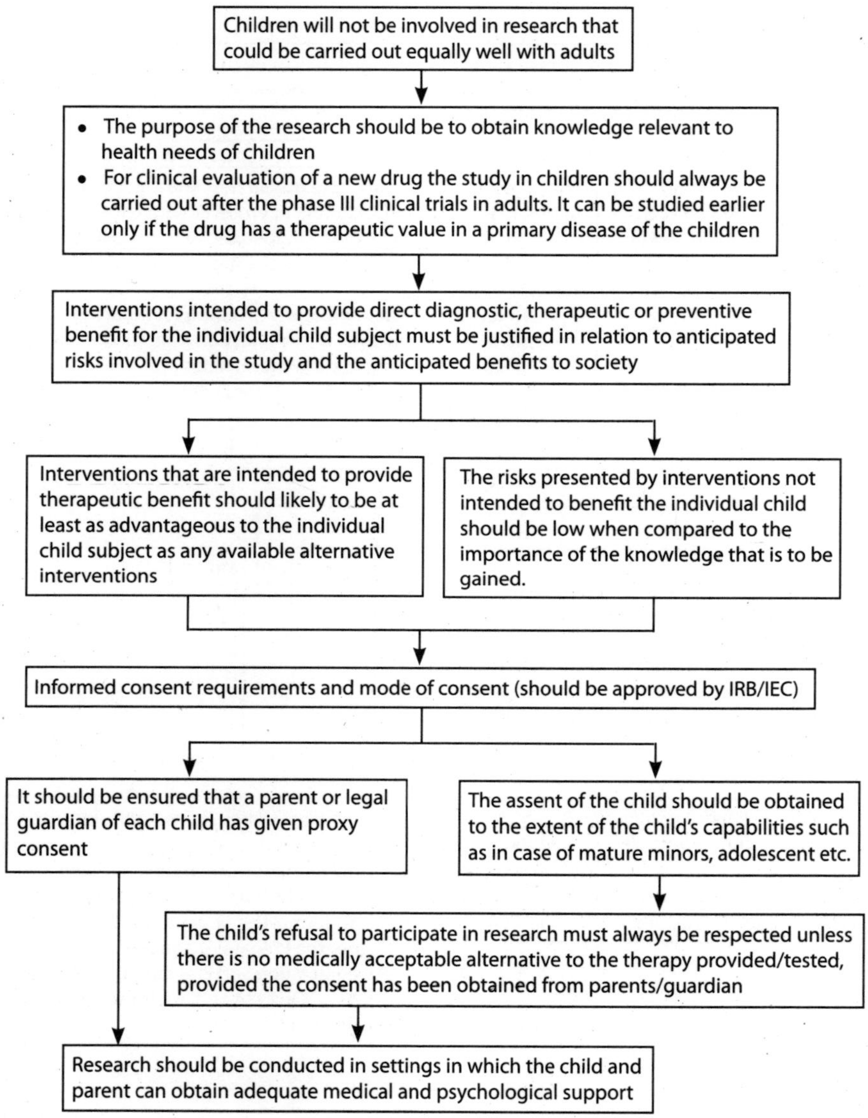

FLOWCHART 11E VULNERABLE SUBJECTS AS RESEARCH SUBJECT

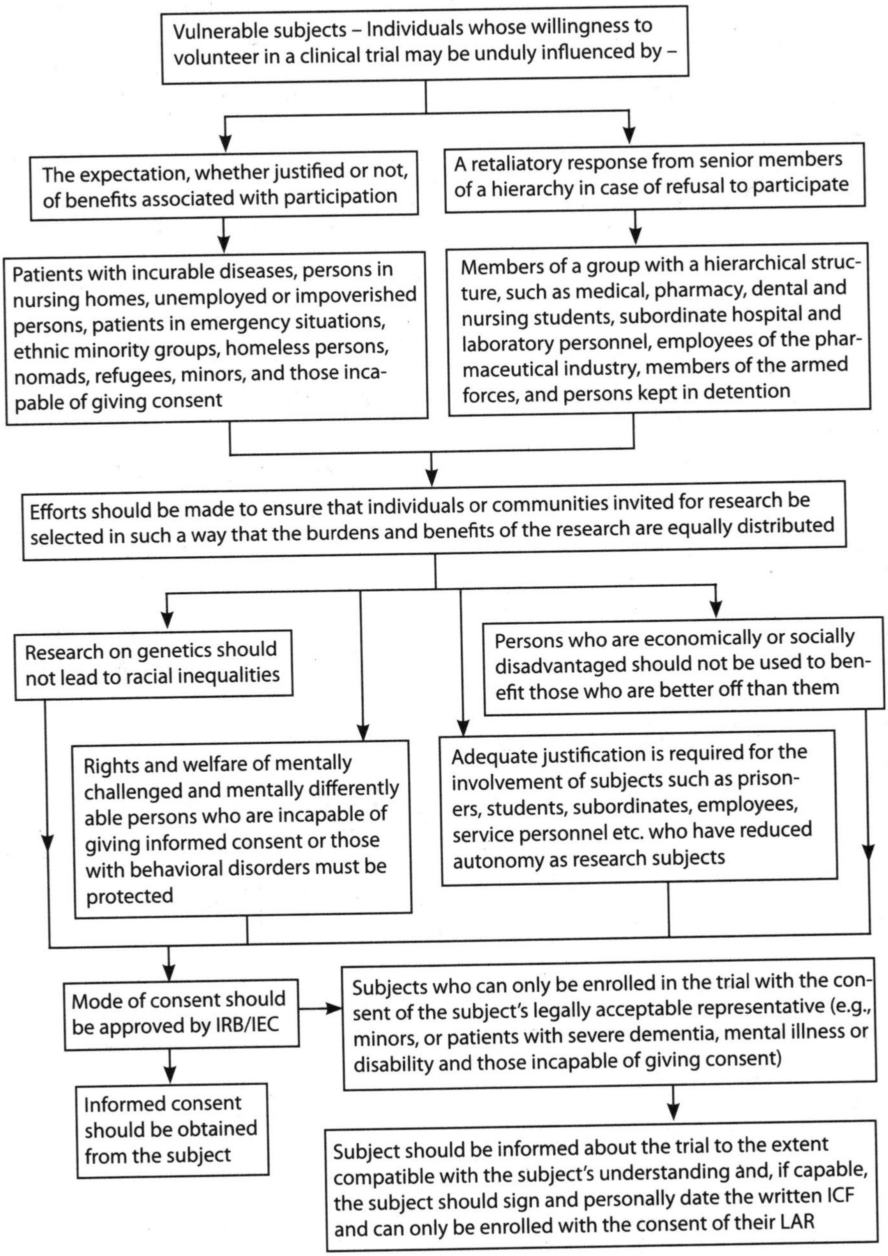

FLOWCHART 12 SCREENING AND TRIAL PROCEDURES INITIATION

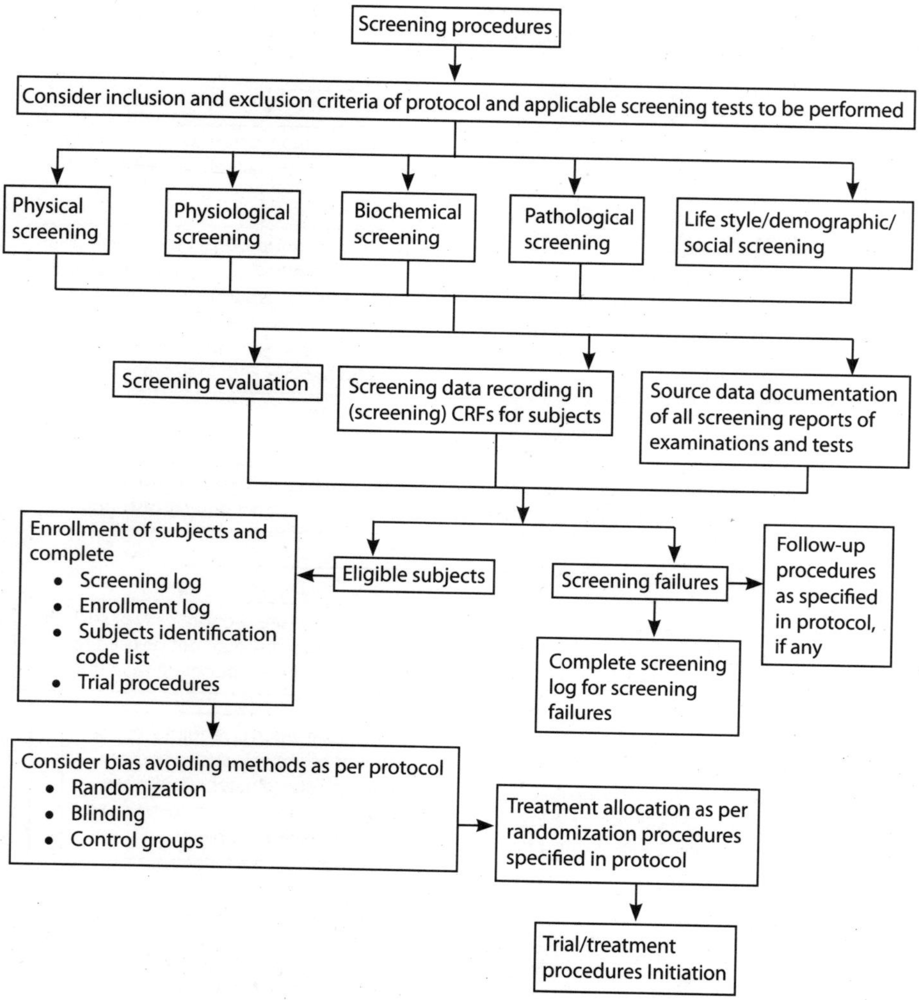

FLOWCHART 13 CLINICAL TRIAL MONITORING

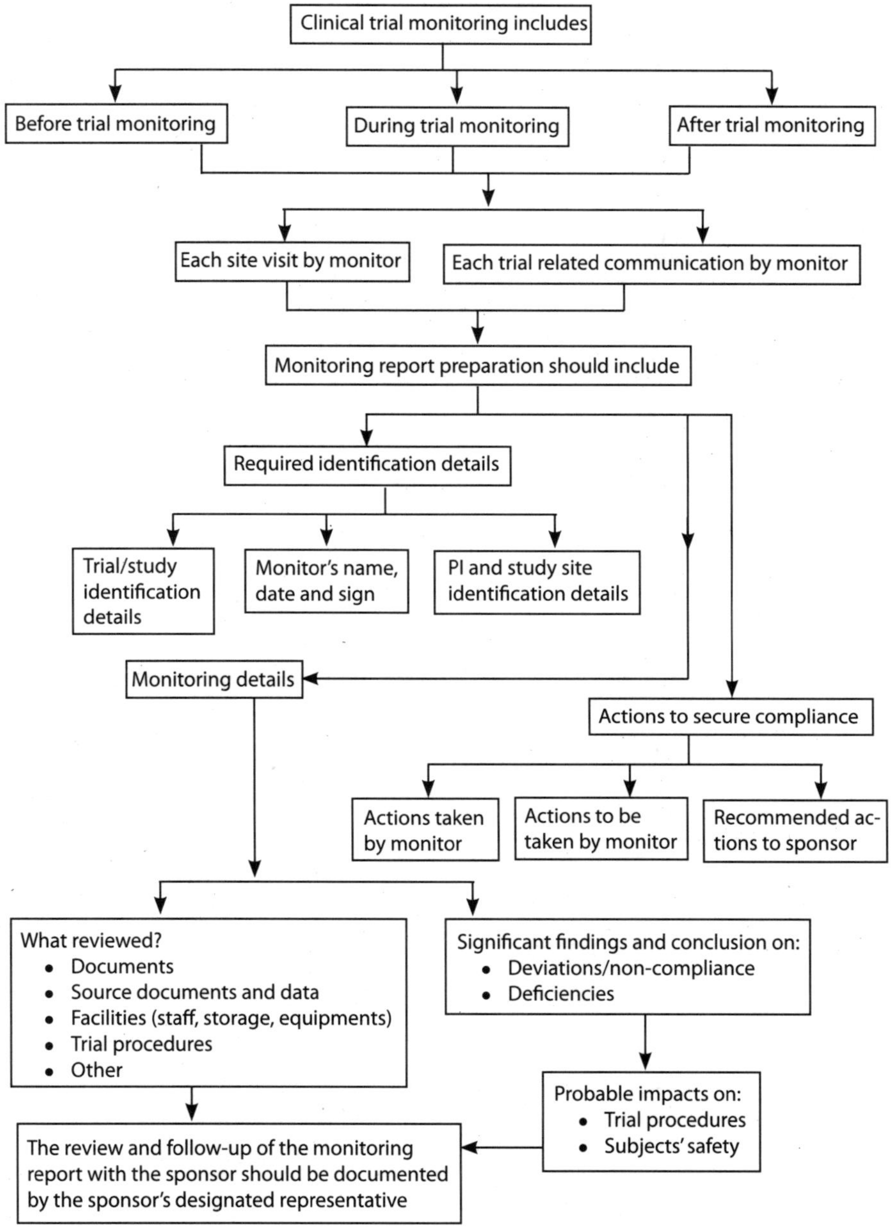

Note: Responsibilities of clinical trial monitor include to ensure that:

- Rights, safety and well being of trial subjects are protected.
- Trial conduct/procedures are in compliance with protocol, GCP and ARRs.
- Reported/recorded data are accurate, complete and verifiable from source documents.

FLOWCHART 14 ONGOING SAFETY EVALUATION AND NEW SAFETY INFORMATION

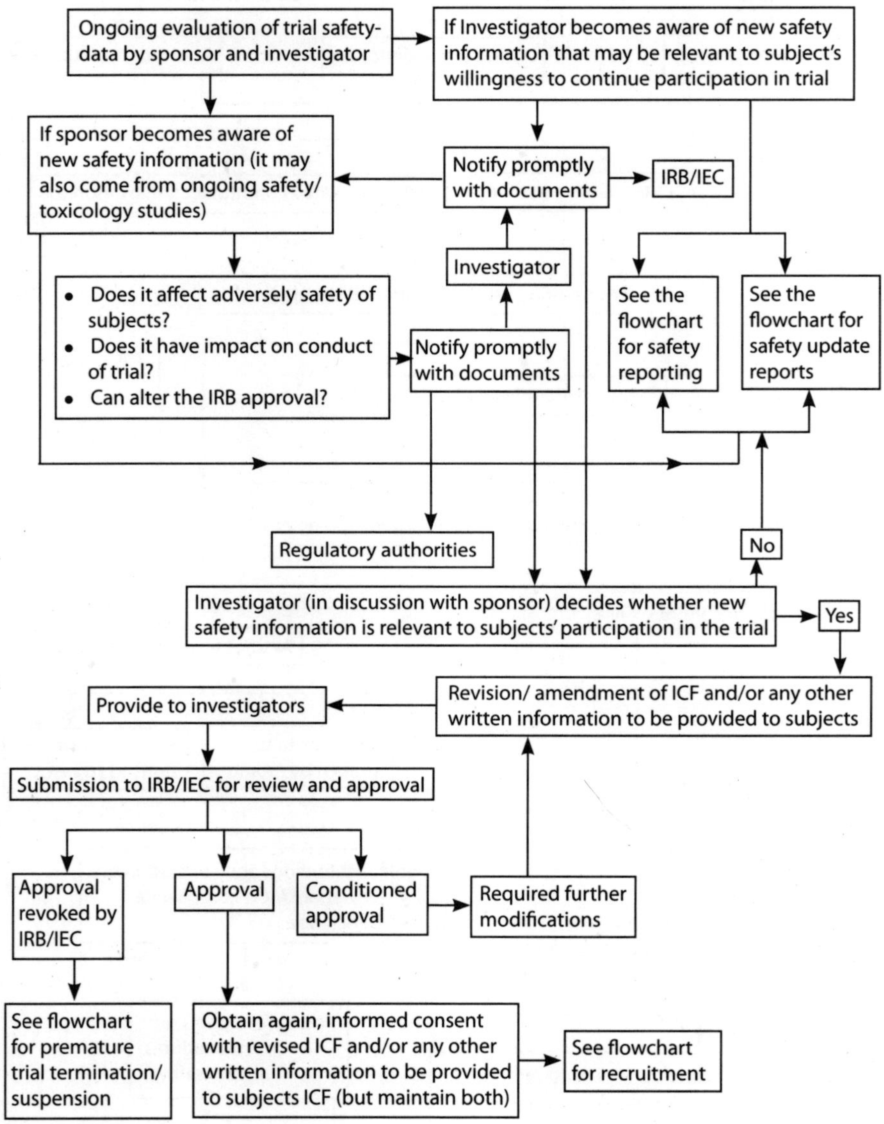

FLOWCHART 15 SAFETY REPORTING

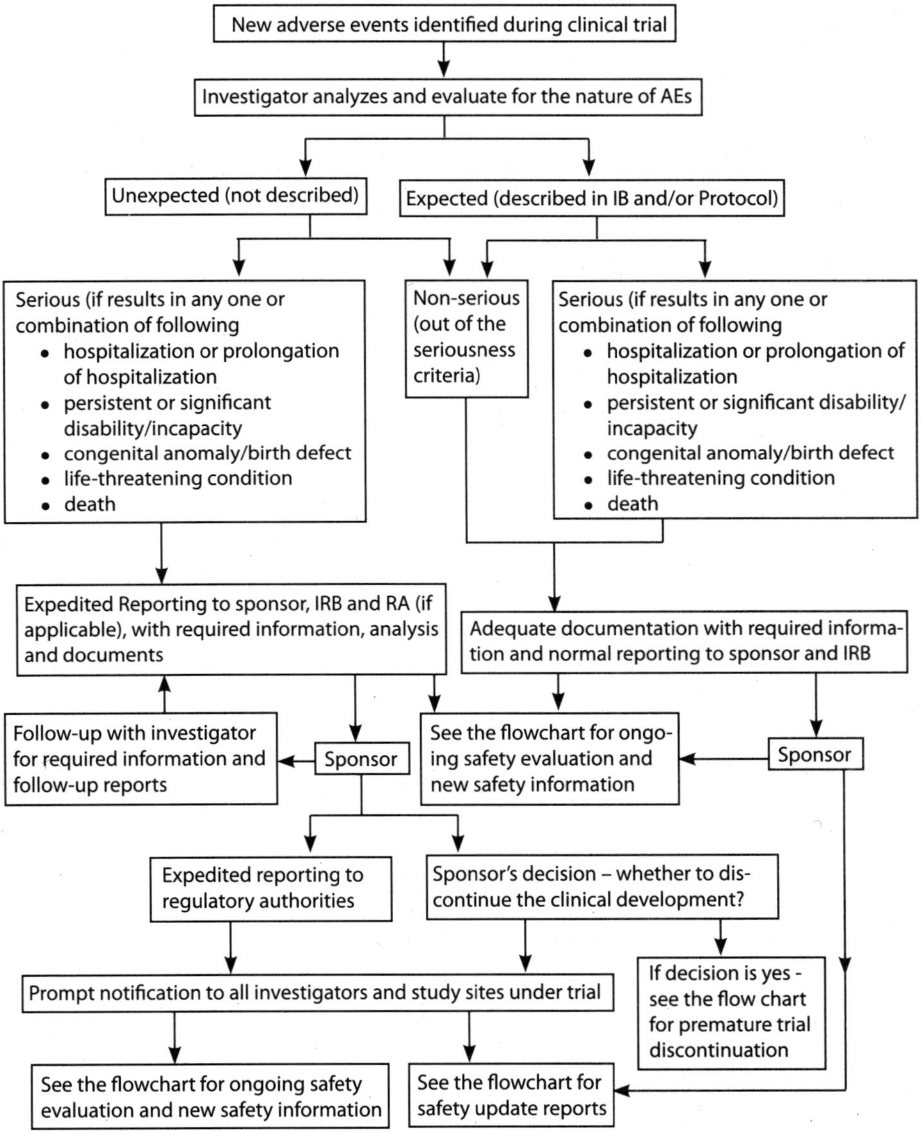

Note: Schedule Y – Investigator shall report all serious and unexpected AEs to sponsor within 24 hours and to EC that accorded approval to the study protocol within 7 working days of their occurrence.

According to Indian GCP, all cases of unexpected and/or SAEs should be reported in expedite manner.

According to Schedule Y, any unexpected SAE should be communicated promptly (within 14 calendar days) by the sponsor to the Licensing Authority and to other investigators participating in the study.

FLOWCHART 16 SAFETY UPDATES REPORTS AND TRIAL PROGRESS REPORTS

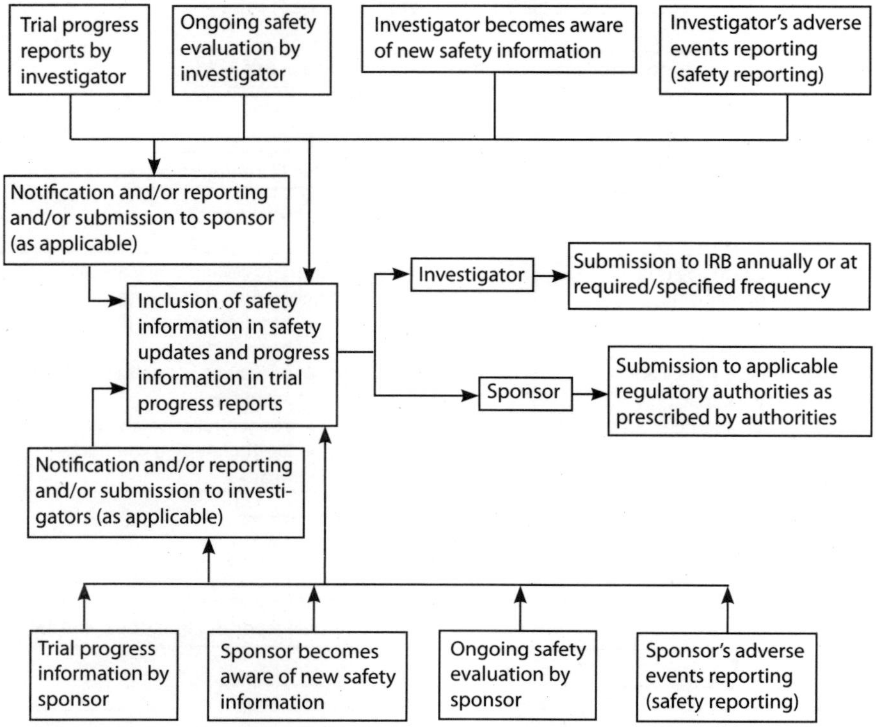

FLOWCHART 17 DEVIATION/NON-COMPLIANCE ON THE PART OF INVESTIGATOR

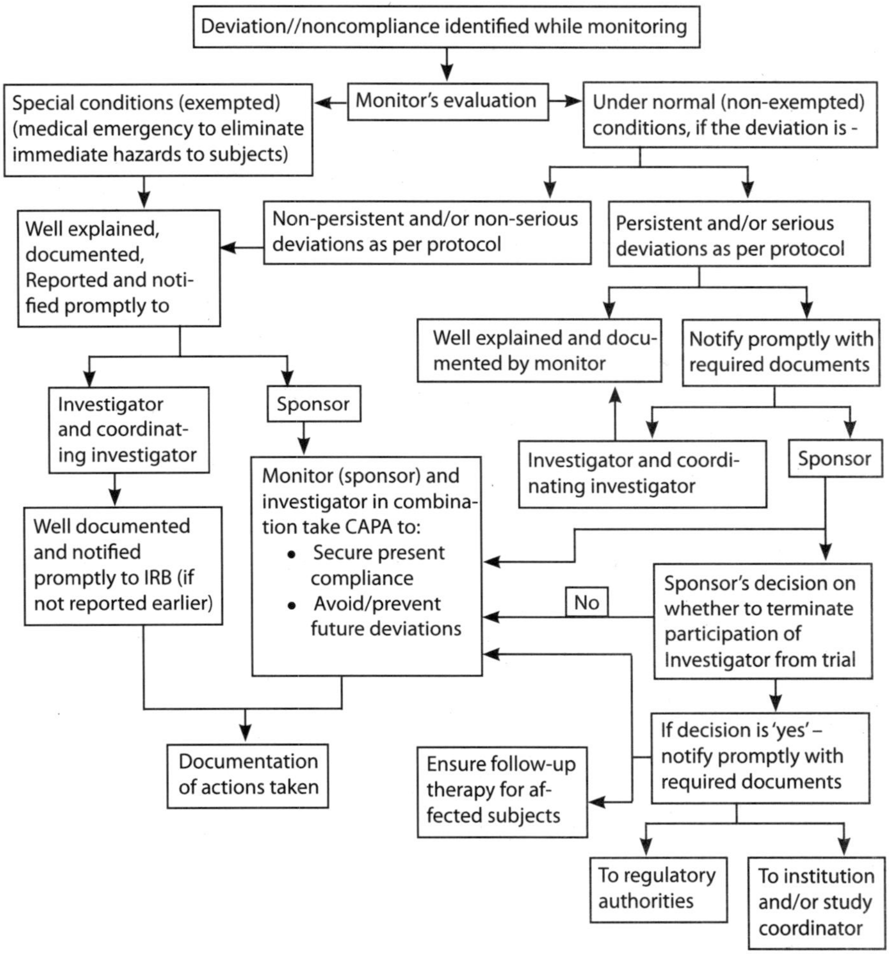

FLOWCHART 18 MODIFICATIONS/AMENDMENTS IN THE STUDY PROTOCOL

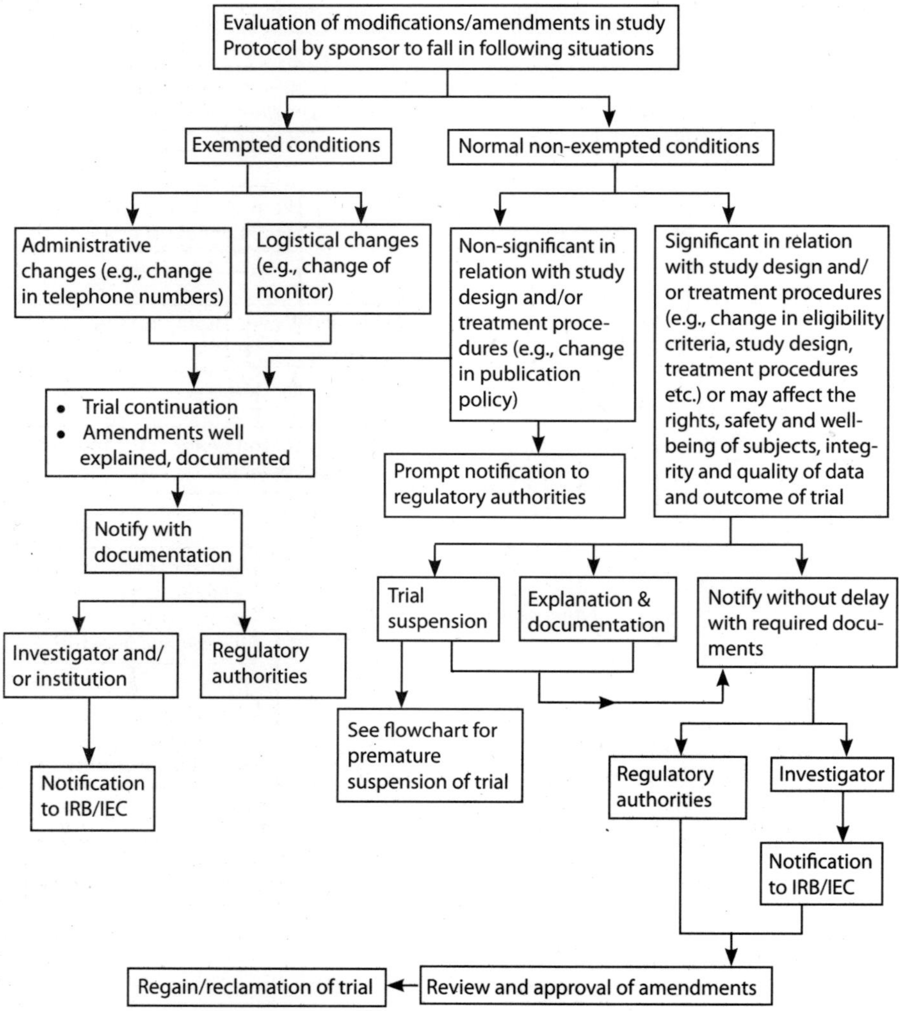

Note: According to Schedule Y, administrative and/or logistic changes in the protocol should be notified to the Licensing Authority within 30 days.

FLOWCHART 19 PREMATURE TERMINATION OR SUSPENSION OF CLINICAL TRIAL

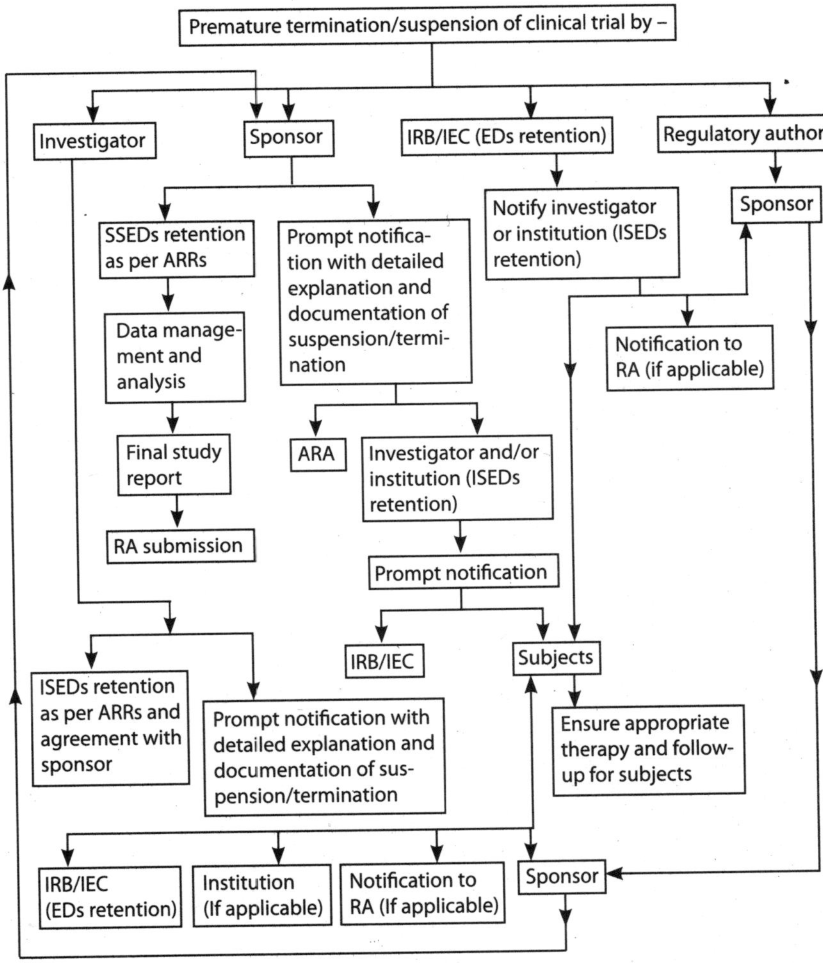

Note: According to Schedule Y, if a study is prematurely discontinued for any reason including lack of commercial interest in pursuing the new drug application, a summary report should be submitted within 3 months.

FLOWCHART 20 TRIAL COMPLETION

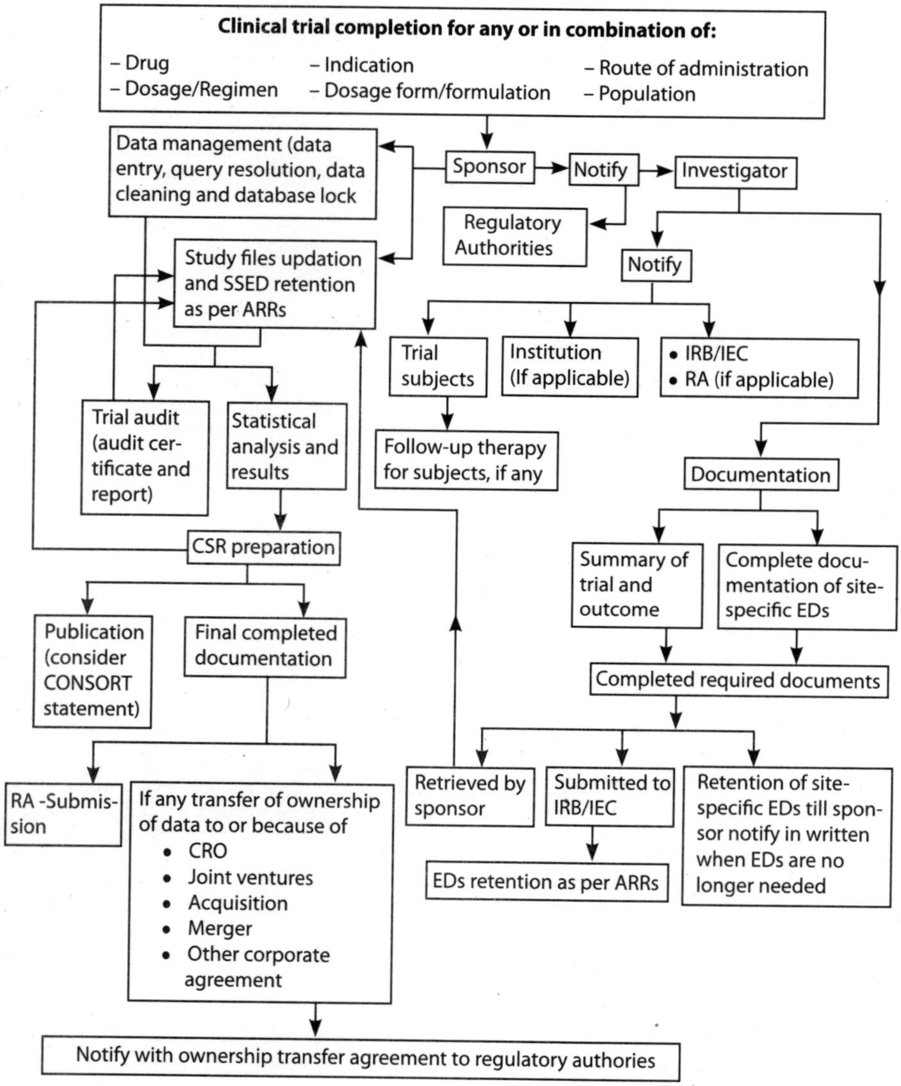

Chapter 4

Miscellaneous Topics in Conduct of Clinical Trials

STAKEHOLDERS IN CLINICAL TRIALS

The key stakeholders in a clinical trial include the following:

- Sponsor (including the monitor, auditor, biostatistician and other trial-related personnel at sponser end)
- Investigation site team (headed by the principal investigator, sub-investigator, pharmacist, nurses, etc.)
- IRB/IEC
- Regulatory Authority/Competent Authority
- Contract Research Organization and other vendor facilities (if contracted by the Sponsor)

STEPS IN CLINICAL TRIAL CONDUCT

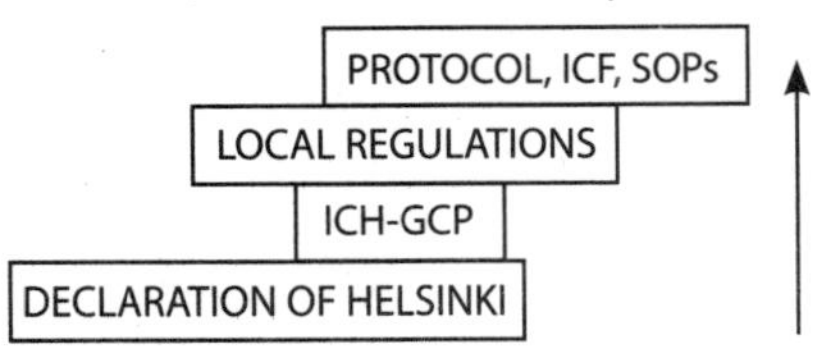

The primary consideration for the conduct of a clinical trial should be the ethical principles of Declaration of Helsinki. Then the ICH-GCP and domestic regulations (i.e., Indian GCP, Schedule Y and ICMR Code)

should be considered. It is recommended that a stringent framework satisfying both global and local regulations be prepared. Based on this framework, the study-related documents and procedures should be designed and defined.

INFORMED CONSENT DOCUMENT

Informed Consent Documents (ICD) include the Informed Consent Form (ICF), where the concerned personnel sign and date, and Patient Information Sheet (PIS), which contains all information regarding the study to be provided to the subject.

INFORMED CONSENT

- For illiterate or blind subjects, impartial witness (IW) is needed.
- If the subject and/or LAR is illiterate, thumb impression should be taken.
- Legally acceptable representatives (LAR) include
  - Parents (by default)
  - If parents are not available, then a judiciary or a relative legally accepted by court/law can be the LAR, i.e. legal custodian.
- In case the subject is a minor and having negative assent but LAR is having positive consent, the patient can be enrolled but negative assent should be recorded, adequately justified and approved by the IRB/IEC with verification from LAR.
- A literate subject can be an IW for another subject if the subject in question agrees.
- An IW should always be a person able to read and understand the contents of ICD well and any other information given to the subject. It is important that the patient/subject in question should agree with the IW. It is preferred that the IW is a LAR (if literate) or a relative of the subject or is well known to the subject.

NATURE OF THE SUBJECT AND NATURE OF THE TRIAL

- Before obtaining the informed consent, the nature of the patient population (e.g., children, vulnerable, pregnant women, etc.) and the nature of the trial (therapeutic or non-therapeutic) should be considered and consent obtained accordingly by taking special measures.

- If the subject comes under more than one category, special care is required in obtaining informed consent. The requirements of informed consent should satisfy all the categories under which the subject falls. The mode of obtaining informed consent should be approved by the IRB/IEC.

RE-CONSENT ISSUES

Informed consent has always been one of the complex processes often closely observed by the auditors and/or inspectors. Once the informed consent is obtained from clinical trial subjects, a re-consent is an important ethical aspect in clinical trials in terms of "when a re-consent should be obtained". However, no clear guidelines are available. It is recommended to divide a typical informed consent process into two parts:

1. Process part
2. Documentation part

If an error has occurred in the process part, it is recommended that re-consent be obtained since a wrong process might jeopardize the rights, safety and welfare of clinical trial subjects. If an error has occurred in the documentation part, re-consenting may not be necessary; however, the error should be rectified satisfactorily with appropriate documentation.

Examples of different types of errors anticipated in the process and documentation parts of informed consent process are:

1. Possible errors in the process part:
   a. When obsolete/wrong/unapproved version of ICF and/or PIS was used.
   b. When inadequate information was provided in ICF and/or PIS.
   c. When language(s) used in ICF and/or PIS is not understandable by the subjects.
   d. LAR and/or IW were required but not present during the informed consent process.
   e. When consent was given by unauthorized persons.

   f. When informed consent process was executed by unauthorized persons.

2. Possible errors in the documentation part:
   a. If date of informed consent is missing in ICF.
   b. When typographical errors occurred in ICF and/or PIS.

Apart from the above errors, there can be other issues that one should pay attention to:

1. The sponsor and/or investigator may became aware of new safety information which can
   a. adversely affect the safety of the subject, or
   b. have impact on the conduct of the trial, or
   c. alter the IRB and/or approval,

   which in turn have impact on the subject's continued participation in the trial, then obtaining re-consent is recommended.
2. To 'dechallenge' or 'rechallenge' medical decisions taken by the investigator in favor of safety of the subjects, re-consent may not be required; however it should be dealt with adequate documentation.

DEVIATIONS, VIOLATIONS AND NON-COMPLIANCE

There is no strict difference in the meanings of these terms. However, some organizations follow the practice of identifying between deviations and violations based on the seriousness involved.

Deviations which may affect the integrity and quality of data generated in clinical trials, as well as the safety, rights and wellbeing of the study subjects and outcomes of the study, are generally referred as violations. For example, if informed consent was not obtained from one or more study subjects, it is regarded an extreme violation of the ethical codes governing the conduct of clinical trials and may have adverse effects on the rights, safety and wellbeing of the subjects concerned.

On the other hand, deviations are minor in nature and do not involve the factors covered for violations. For example, if the monitor during a visit forgets to sign on the monitoring log at the trial site, it is regarded as deviation from "monitoring SOP".

In literary terms, these all have same meaning, implying that something has gone wrong and needs to be corrected. However, no generalization should be made as to deviations are always minor, violations are major and non-compliance is acting against the applicable regulations. It all depends on "related or against to what". One should speak "in relation to what", e.g., deviation/violation against a protocol; deviation/violation against a specific SOP; deviation/violation against a GCP; or deviation/violation against the applicable regulatory requirements.

UNIDENTIFIABLE OR NON-ASSESSABLE ADVERSE EVENTS

If during the course of a clinical trial any adverse event is reported for which any or all of the following elements cannot be identified or assessed at the time of reporting:

- Seriousness
- Causal relationship with IP
- Expectedness or unexpectedness

It is recommended to treat these AEs as suspected events for the above parameters. For example, if a woman reports pregnancy during the course of a trial, the investigator may not be able to assess the effects of study interventions on the fetus. Therefore, it is recommended that pregnancy should be considered as serious adverse event because, later, it may fall within the criteria of seriousness, i.e. congenital birth defect/anomaly.

MUST THE INVESTIGATOR BE A PHYSICIAN?

The FDA regulations do not require that the investigator be a physician. However, sponsors are required to select only investigators who are qualified, trained and experienced to investigate the drug. In case the clinical investigator is a non-physician, a qualified physician (or dentist, when appropriate) should be listed as a sub-investigator and should be responsible for all trial-related medical (or dental) decisions (ICH E6 section 4.3.1).

ICH-GCP further states that the investigator should be qualified, trained and experienced to assume responsibility for the proper conduct of a trial, and should meet all the qualifications specified by the applicable regulatory requirements, whereas Indian GCP states that the investigator should have qualifications prescribed by the Medical Council of India (MCI).

RAW DATA OR SOURCE DATA/DOCUMENTS

Both terms have a similar meaning. Source documents are those documents where the data related to trial subjects and their treatment procedures were entered for the first time.

"ALCOA" PRINCIPLE FOR SOURCE DATA

Source data are the data recorded on source documents. Source data in a clinical trial should have the following properties.

- **Attributable**

  The source data should be attributed to the person recording it. All source data captured should be signed by the person recording it.

- **Legible**

  The source data should be in a readable, comprehensible, understandable language.

- **Contemporaneous**

  The source data should be recorded at the same time of the occurrence of an event or activity. A clear date should be indicated. This should help the auditor/monitor to reconstruct the series of events that occurred at different points of time.

- **Original**

  The source data present on file should be original for the sake of verification. In case if any photocopies are present, the same should be authenticated by the investigator or authorized personnel as in the authorization log.

- **Accurate**

  The source data should be true, correct and precise and the same should be recorded on the CRFs. The transcription of data from source to CRFs should be accurate.

PROTOCOL

- It is preferred to take KOL's inputs and opinions for protocol writing.

- Protocol amendments
  - If minor – notification is enough (e.g., administrative and logistic changes)
  - If major – prior approval before implementation is required

INVESTIGATOR'S BROCHURE

- While designing and compiling it, one should think for the perspective that: "shall the PI accept this treatment or IB for their patients?"
- IB objective – should be non-promotional since it has a research purpose
- Editing and formatting of IB should be such that the PI can understand it better
  - Editing should be preferably done by medically qualified persons
- As clinical development progresses (considerations for IB are)
  - Data on non/pre-clinical studies gets abbreviated
  - Data of effects on humans gets on populating
- IB is not needed to be approved by IRB but it is required to obtain necessary information on IP.

CASE REPORT FORM (CRF)

- CRF is designed based on protocols keeping in mind that all the necessary data are captured into appropriate sections of CRF.
- In NCR (no carbon required) CRFs, it is suggested to have 3 copies of each page (one each for PI, sponsor and data entry/ management).
- Data which is required to be transcribed from source documents on to CRF should never be recorded directly on CRF unless it is specified in the approved study protocol. In case if some data is being recorded directly on to the CRF, then the CRF will be considered as a source document for such data.
- Electronic archival should be done with a data reader instrument (since technologies keep changing with time, a data reader instrument may not be available at the time of data review).

IRB/IEC

- In case one IRB has rejected the study protocol and the sponsor is seeking approval from another IRB, then the sponsor should intimate the latter regarding the earlier protocol refusal with reasons stated by the previous IRB.

REVIEWS BY IRB/IEC

Three types of review (for the study proposal) may be conducted by an IRB/IEC.

- Initial review – these reviews are conducted when a new study proposal is submitted to an IRB/IEC for the purpose of taking a decision whether to approve or not, or to suggest required modifications for approval.
- Interim/ongoing/periodic reviews – these reviews are conducted at appropriate time intervals as stipulated in the SOP of IRB/IEC which should be indicated to the investigator and/or sponsor.
- Conditioned/case review – these reviews are conducted when need arises (e.g., major protocol amendment or new information that may influence the conduct or outcomes of the study and/or rights, safety and wellbeing of study subjects).

AUDIT

- Auditors are independent of the conduct of the trial
  - Independent of PI/site/trial
  - However, may not be independent of the sponsor (i.e., may be sponsor's personnel who is/are not involved in the trial or sometimes external auditor may be contracted).
- Audit should verify that the trial is being or has been conducted actually by ICF verification.
- The auditor verifies the compliance of trial-related activities and reports non-compliance or deviation, if found, whereas the monitor verifies the compliance, reports any non-compliance or deviation, and ensures compliance by corrective actions with PI and sponsor.

CLINICAL TRIALS REGISTRY OF INDIA (CTRI)

The Clinical Trials Registry of India (CTRI) was set up by the ICMR's National Institute of Medical Statistics (NIMS) and is funded by the Department of Science and Technology (DST) through the Indian Council of Medical Research (ICMR). It also receives financial and technical support through the WHO-SEARO (WHO-South-East Asia Regional Office) and the WHO India Country office.

CTRI is an online register of clinical trials being conducted in India. Any researcher who plans to conduct a trial involving human participants is expected to register the trial in CTRI before enrollment of the first participant. A sponsor should voluntarily disclose the details of clinical trial to the CTRI. CTRI is a part of ICMR and is one of the primary register of the WHO. The main objective of CTRI is to ensure free availability of information regarding clinical trials conducted in India; thereby ensuring transparency, accountability and accessibility of clinical trials and their results. The CTRI dataset and requirements for CTRD (Clinical Trial Registry Database) and registration of clinical trials are available at http://www.ctri.in/Clinicaltrials/CTRI_Dataset_and_Description.doc.

COMMON GCP ISSUES DURING THE TRIAL/STUDY

Below are highlighted some common issues which if remain non-compliant to the GCP may raise a concern/question regarding the validity of the clinical trial. These issues require more attention to prevent any non-compliance.

Informed Consent

- Correct (approved) version should be used for obtaining informed consent.
- Copy of ICF and PIS should be provided to the patients.
- Documentation of subject's contacts/identity should be done only in source documents to maintain confidentiality of trial subjects' identity.
- Properly translated ICF, if required, should be used to obtain informed consent.
- Impartial witness and/or LAR, if required, should be involved during informed consent process.

Recruitment and Study Procedures

- Screening for trial subjects should be done always after obtaining informed consent.
- All protocols indicated/required laboratory tests/investigations should be conducted for trial subjects.
- Eligibility should be proven for trial subjects entering into the clinical trial as per the inclusion/exclusion criteria.
- Advertisements used for subject recruitment should be approved by the ethics committee.

Monitoring

- Verification of data transcribed from source documents to the CRF should be done.
- The data recorded on CRF should be of acceptable quality and complete in all respects.
- All the necessary documents should be properly documented and retained in the study files.
- The frequency of monitoring (agreed between the sponsor and regulatory authorities) should be implemented as specified in the protocol.

Clinical Trial Supplies

- For randomized clinical trials, errors in assigning randomization codes should be avoided by adequate review.
- Complete IP accountability should be documented at the trial site.
- IP should be stored at the trial site as specified in the IB or protocol.
- Blind-breaking procedures should be designed and implemented in such a way that it should not have any effect on the data, subjects and outcomes of the trial.

Safety Information

- Some SAEs remain unreported or reported with delay to the regulatory authorities and IRB/IEC because of the deficient system of collecting information, tracking and follow-up. Adequate system should be implemented for identifying, recording, reporting and following-up of SAEs.

- All AEs and SAEs should be adequately documented in the source documents as well.
- Failure in obtaining additional informed consent in an ongoing trial in case any new safety information is observed during the trial which may jeopardize or change the safety or decision of trial subjects to continue participating in the trial.
- Timely updating of the IB for observed AEs and/or SAEs as per the implemented SOP.
- New relevant safety information, if identified during the trial, should be transmitted to all participating investigators in a multicentre study.

INQUIRY BY REGULATORY AUTHORITIES

During an inspection visit, regulatory authorities usually inquire about the following issues. The main concern of regulatory authorities includes the safety of patients, ethical standards of trial and the integrity and quality of the trial data.

- Source of study subjects (e.g. patient population at study site or advertisement)
- Did the patients have the disease under investigation at the time of enrollment?
- Did the trial subjects meet the eligibility criteria?
- Was the protocol followed precisely?
- Were AEs and SAEs reported appropriately?

COMMON FINDINGS IN A REGULATORY INSPECTION

The common findings are as given below. These require special attention and should be rectified well before the inspection.

- Failure to adhere to protocol specifications which may include the following:
  - Disparities between the patient's screening status and the eligibility criteria.
  - Errors in the randomized allocation of trial subjects.
  - Some tests not conducted for one or more trial subjects.

   - Changes in the subjects' treatment not authorized by the sponsor or not approved by regulatory authorities and/or IEC/IRB.
- Failure to maintain adequate/accurate records which may include the following:
   - Any change in trial data with proper justification.
   - One or more records destroyed or missing.
   - Failure of accurate data recording on all trial-related documents specifically the source documents and CRFs.
- Failure to report concomitant therapies administered to the trial subjects.
- Failure to maintain complete IP accountability records.
- Failure to obtain proper informed consent as per the regulations.
- IRB failed to review the research at a convened meeting.
- Investigators fail to report promptly unanticipated problems involving risks to subjects or IRB/IEC and/or sponsor.
- Proposed ongoing review/evaluation of research/safety information was not substantial and meaningful.
- IRB did not ensure additional protection to vulnerable subjects.
- IRB members inappropriately participated in new and continuing reviews of protocols of which they had conflicting interest.

INVESTIGATOR-SPONSORED TRIAL (IST)

Investigator-sponsored trials are those in which the investigator and the sponsor for the trial is one and same. For example, if a physician on his/her own conducts a trial in his/her clinical settings with the responsibilities of both an investigator and a sponsor, it is regarded an IST and the investigator is responsible to follow the regulations and guidelines. Globally and in India too, many ISTs are performed by one or more investigators as a team and usually initiated by research hospitals.

Generally the aim of ISTs conducted by physicians is to publish the trial findings. However, one or more pharmaceutical companies can be involved as financing and supporting agency but they may not be responsible for violations to the regulations and guidelines.

These studies sometimes are also referred as "investigator-initiated trials".

APPLICABLE REGULATORY AUTHORITIES (ARA)

Applicable regulatory authorities are those regulatory agencies to whom the stakeholders of clinical trials are responsible for designing, conducting and reporting a clinical trial. There may be one or more ARAs for a trial. For example, if any sponsor conducts a clinical trial in India with the intention to submit the data also to FDA (trial initiated with FDA approval in addition to DCGI approval), then both DCG(I) and FDA will be the ARA. A national regulatory authority in a country where the trial is being conducted always comes under ARAs, and the clinical trial should be compliant with the regulations of that national regulatory authority. Finally, a report of the trial is required to be submitted to that national regulatory authority. Furthermore, if a trial is global is nature with the intention to obtain approval in more than one country, then all the regulatory authorities of the intended/targeted countries and the regulatory authority of the country where the trial is being conducted will come under the ARAs, provided prior approvals have been taken from all the regulatory authorities from whom the sponsor is planning to get approval for the drug. In short, we can say that all the regulatory authorities who have given approval for a clinical trial in question will come under the applicable regulatory authorities. Some of the regulatory authorities of different countries or regions are mentioned below.

- DCG(I) – India
- FDA – United States of America
- MHRA – United Kingdom
- MHLW – Japan
- EMEA – Europe
- MCC – South Africa
- TGA – Australia
- TPD – Canada
- ANVISA – Brazil

"GCP tells
What to do but not
How to do."

Chapter 5

Quality, Compliance and Management Issues

Achieving and maintaining good compliance and quality in clinical trials is the shared responsibility of each individual and stakeholder involved, and is a challenge rather than an operation. Quality, compliance and project management are three most important factors determining the reliability of data and successful completion of a clinical trial.

- Quality can be defined as a measure of excellence or state of being free from defects, deficiencies or significant variations from predetermined parameters and standards.
- Compliance may be defined as adherence of trial related activities and procedures with applicable regulatory requirements.
- Project management is the application of knowledge, skills, tools and techniques into the project in order to meet or exceed stakeholder's expectations from a project.

With reference to clinical trials, these three terms are highly interrelated and have the potential to influence other parameters as well, and hence they need to be dealt with in combination. The term "Quality System" is preferred by the author to combine quality, compliance and project management, and it is expected the readers have no confusion between the terms quality and quality system. We discuss the Quality System under the following heads:

(a) Establishment of the Quality System

(b) Implementation of the Quality System

(c) Control and Evaluation of the Quality System

(d) Updating the Quality System

ESTABLISHMENT OF THE QUALITY SYSTEM

Project Planning

Planning plays an important role in the success of clinical trials. A well-planned study project is valuable in terms of cost, time, resources, etc. A clinical trial should be properly planned by the project manager, and an overall project plan should be prepared with acceptable flexibility to meet unforeseen future conditions. An overview of project planning is provided in the chapter "Clinical Trial Framework".

Human Resource Planning and Establishment

Before a clinical trial project begins, the sponsor should make available adequate human resources. For successful running of a clinical trial project, the following personnel may be required.

Designation	Chief Role
Project Manager (PM)	Facilitator, Manager
Clinical Research Associate (CRA)	Liaison with investigators, assist PM with project administration
Clinical Research Monitor (CRM)	Site monitoring as per ICH GCP
Site Coordinators	Coordinate activities on site
Medical Advisors	Determine medical data to be collected
Manufacturing Specialist	Supervise manufacturing and delivery of drug materials
Biostatistician	Trial design including the determination of sample size and method of analysis
Regulatory Liaison	Liaison with regulatory agencies
Marketing Liaison	Assist in project feasibility assessment and planning
Attorney	Draft all legal agreements
Technical/Medical Writers	For preparing CSR, ASR, PSUR, IB and other medical documents
Lead Programmers (LP)	Develop data entry and handling system
Database Manager	Integrity and security of data
Data Management Personnel	Data management activities

Quality Assurance and Quality Control Planning and Establishment

1. Standard Operating Procedures (SOPs) should be established for important activities and functions to be carried out in a clinical trial involving all ethical, regulatory and sponsor's requirements. These SOPs can be categorized into sections concerning the sponsor, monitor and investigator site.

   The list of important SOPs given below is based on major activities in a clinical trial. The list may not be exhaustive and depends on practices being followed by individual clinical trial stakeholders. In the list given below, monitor, CRO and similar facilities have been considered as part of sponsor's responsibilities. However, if few activities or responsibilities have been delegated to vendors (outsourced), these facilities may have their specific SOPs as agreed upon by the concerned parties. To ensure compliance, quality and project management, vendor audit may be performed.

Table 1 SOPs to be Established for Clinical Trials

S.No.	Activities Requiring SOPs
	Sponsor's SOPs
1	Preparation, review and amendments of protocol
2	Preparation, review and updating of investigator's brochure
3	Preparation, review, amendments and translation of informed consent form
4	Preparation and updating of clinical database
5	Clinical database entry procedures
6	Data clarification, cleaning and locking procedures
7	IP management (packaging, coding, labeling of IP(s) containers and sample retention and deficient product recall)
8	Shipment and disposition of IP(s)
9	Preparation, updating and retention of study files and documents
10	Procedures for breaking of blind
11	Vendor audit procedures (e.g. for CRO, logistics, data management facility, if outsourced)
12	Preparation and implementation of agreements with other parties involved in the trial
13	Conducting trial site evaluation visits
14	Conducting site initiation visits
15	Conducting monitoring visits
16	Conducting site close-out visits
17	Conduction of clinical trials audits
18	Identifying, analyzing and reporting of safety information
19	Premature study site or trial suspension and termination
20	Preparing clinical study reports
	Investigator Site's SOPs
1	Obtaining IRB approval
2	Obtaining informed consent from study subjects
3	IP management at site (receipt, handling, storage, dispensing, retrieval, accountability & disposition)
4	Recording and retention of study files and documents
5	Identifying, analyzing and reporting of safety information
6	Preparing Interim and final trial progress/summary reports
7	Follow-up procedures after the trial

2. The formats of principal documents of a clinical trial (Protocol, IB, ICF and CRF) should be standardized with applicable ethical guidelines, GCP, applicable regulatory requirements and interests of the sponsor company.
3. Standard formats for data capturing, reporting, documentation-related activities and notifications should be established in correspondence with sponsor, GCP and applicable regulatory requirements. These can be treated as attachment forms and reports for applicable SOPs.
4. Prior to initiating a clinical trial, Monitoring Plan and Audit Plan should be prepared identifying the purpose, extent, nature and required frequency of monitoring and audit in addition to procedures describing what, when and how to review.
5. A data handling system should be designed by the sponsor with the following requirements:
   - Completeness
   - Reliability
   - Consistency
   - Accuracy
   - Maintaining audit trail
   - Security and avoiding unauthorized access
   - Adequate back-up of data
   - Safeguard of blinding, randomization etc.

Resources Planning and Establishment

The sponsor should ensure adequate resource availability prior to and throughout the entire course of the clinical trial.

Such resources include printers, computers, photocopiers, internet and intranet facility, communication portals, IP storage and shipment/transport facility, facility for document archiving and retention, etc. For effective resource planning, the sponsor should identify sequential needs at different steps in a clinical trial.

Budgetary Planning

Budgetary planning implies the forecasting of anticipated monetary expenses for each individual activity as well as for the whole trial collectively. The sponsor should analyze trial activities individually to forecast the associated future cost for smooth running of the trial. Below is given a format with arbitrary values for cost estimations of trial-related activities, which may be used to develop a budgetary plan for a typical study. The number and type of study-related activities depend on the nature of study, availability of resources and sponsor-specific requirements.

Proposed Budget

Investigational Product: CETUXIMAB An open label, multinational, randomized, controlled trial in metastatic colorectal cancer Number of patients, n = 450 at 20 sites (10 in India, 10 abroad)				
S. No	**Heads**	**Calculation**	**Total (INR in Lakhs)**	**Assumption**
A	**Site Expenses**			
1	Patient day care charges	10000 x 450 x 4	180.00	10000/pt for 4 visits
2	Patient hospitalization charges	50000 x 225	113.00	50000/pt assuming hospitalization for SAEs for 50% pts during the study
3	Institutional charges	(180 + 112.5) x 20/100	59.00	Assuming 20% of total hospitalization and day care charges
4	Telecom charges	2000 x 10 x 24 + 5000 x 10 x 24	17.00	2000/month/Indian site and 5000/month/abroad site for ~ 24 months
5	Central lab charges	10000 x 450 x 4 + 10000 x 300	210.00	10000/patient/visit, and 300 unscheduled visits
6	Charges for radiological investigations	25000 x 6 x 450	675.00	25000/investigation/patient and 6 investigations/patient
7	Total investigation charges for screen failures	(25000 + 10000) x 100	35.00	(assuming 100 screen failures) lab and radiological investigations
8	EC Fee including review fees	30000 x 10 + 50000 x 10	8.00	10 sites in India (30000/EC) and 10 sites abroad (50000/EC)
9	Investigator Fee	100000 x 450	450.00	100000/pt for whole study
Total Site Expenses 1747.00				
B	**Sponsor Expenses**			
10	Regulatory expenses		10.00	Including expenses for fee for regulatory agencies, import authorities, expenses for agents and other resources like telephone, courier etc.
11	Investigator meeting	80 x 120000	100.00	Investigators, co-investigators = 40, study coordinators = 20, sponsor representatives = 10; CRO representative = 10 (Total = 80); Travel and lodging @ 120000/person + other expenses (food, conference, transport etc)

Contd...

12	Drug shipment charges	50000 x 10 x 4 + 100000 x 10 x 4	60.00	50000/consignment (Indian sites) and 100000/consignment (abroad sites); first initial consignment followed by approx 3 more consignments per site
13	PSSV/SEV	20000 x 10 + 100000 x 10	12.00	20000/person for domestic sites and 100000/person for sites abroad
14	SIV	40000 x 10 + 200000 x 10	24.00	40000/site/2 persons for domestic sites and 200000/site/2 persons for sites abroad
15	SMV	20000 x 10 x 5 + 100000 x 10 x 5	60.00	5 visits/ site (frequency of monitoring visits should be derived from the monitoring plan for study)
16	Visits by project manager	20000 x 10 x 2 + 100000 x 10 x 2	24.00	2 visits/site
17	SCV	20000 x 10 x 2 + 100000 x 10 x 2	24.00	2 persons/site
18	Unplanned visit	20000 x 10 x 2 + 100000 x 10 x 2	24.00	2 visits/site
19	CRF printing charges	1000 x 150 + 2000 x 500	12.00	1000/screening CRF; 2000/ Treatment CRF (50 additional copies required of both)
20	ICD translation and printing charges	15000 x 10 + 25000 x 10	4.00	15000/Indian language and 25000/Foreign language; (10 Indian languages + 10 foreign languages
21	CTM courier charges	10000 x 10 x 4 + 50000 x 10 x 4	24.00	10000/courier (Indian sites) and 50000/courier (abroad sites); First initial courier followed by approx 3 more courier/site
22	Clinicaltrial insurance		50.00	Arbitrary assumption
Total Sponsor Expenses 428.00				
C	**Outsourcing Expenses**			
23	CRO/data management and biostatistics		300.00	Arbitrary assumption
Total Outsourcing Expenses 300.00				
D	**Other Expenses**			
24	Infrastructure cost	100000 x 20	20.00	Deep freezer, centrifuge, thermohygrometer, almirah etc. (100000/site)
25	Contingency Budget		20.00	Assumption
26	Investigational Drug Cost		3519.00	(See below the method of drug cost estimation)

Contd...

27	Comparator Drug Cost		3519.00	For ease assumed as similar of investigational drug however it depends on - Comparator drug used and - Dosage and administration schedule
Total Other Expenses 7078.00				
Total expenses 9553.00 **Overhead expenses (10% assumption) 955.30 (~ 2 lakhs per patient)** **Grand Total 10508.00**				

Assumptions

- Number of patients $n = 450$ at 20 sites (10 in India, 10 abroad); approx 23 patients per site
- Sites = 10 in India, 5 in middle east and eastern Europe, and 5 in US and Europe
- Radiological investigations (CT, MRI, etc. for chest, abdomen and pelvis) to be done at baseline, remaining visits and follow-up with a total of 6 investigations/patient.

Note

- Some of these expenses may not be required for trials subjected to the policies and procedures of the sponsor, and some expenses may be required additionally subjected to the need of the study or sponsor policies, e.g. GCP training for site, vendor audits, site audits, managing inspections, etc. Some other considerations may also be required additionally, e.g. cost of withdrawal and dropouts and expenses for the establishment, meetings and consultations of the data monitoring committee.
- Arbitrary cost estimations of the investigational drug
  1. Dosage and administration schedule:
     - Initial dose is 400 mg/m^2 administered one week prior to the initiation of a course of radiation therapy as a 120-minute intravenous infusion
     - Subsequent weekly dose (all other infusions) is 250 mg/m^2 infused over 60-minutes for the duration of radiation therapy (6 weeks)
  2. Presentation of Cituximab
     - 200 mg/100 ml single-use vial and 100 mg/50 ml single-use vial

3. Cost of Cituximab vials (arbitrary)
   - 100 ml vial = \$800
   - 50 ml vial = \$400
4. Average body surface area (BSA) = 1.73 m^2 (assuming adult patients)
5. Initial dose required for one patient = 400 × 1.73 = 692 mg
   - Vials required for initial dose/patient = three 100 ml vials + two 50 ml vials
6. Subsequent individual doses required for one patient = 250 × 1.73 = 433 mg
   - Vials required for a single subsequent dose = two 100 ml vials + one 50 ml vial
   - Total vials needed for all 6 subsequent doses/patient = twelve 100 ml vials + six 50 ml vials
7. Total number of vials required/patient for the whole study = fifteen 100 ml vials + eight 50 ml vials
8. Total vials needed for 450 patients = 450 × 15 (100 ml vials) + 450 × 8 (50 ml vials) = 6750 (100 ml vials) + 3600 (50 ml vials)
9. Contingency requirement = 600 (100 ml vials) + 200 (50 ml vials)
10. Vials required for retention (assumption) = 300 (100 ml vials) + 300 (50 ml vials)
11. Vials required for analysis (assumption) = 50 (100 ml vials) + 50 (50 ml vials)
12. Total requirement for the study = (6750 + 600 + 300 + 50) 100 ml vials and (3600 + 200 + 300 + 50) 50 ml vials = 7700 (100 ml vials) and 4150 (50 ml vials)
13. Total cost for the study of the investigational drug = \$800 × 7700 + \$400 × 4150 = \$6160000 + \$1660000 = \$7820000 = 351900000 INR (assuming conversion factor of 45) = Rs 3519 lakhs

Time Frame Planning

Time frame planning implies the forecasting of time required for the accomplishment of each activity of the clinical trial and trial as a whole.

Forecasting the timelines requires a rigorous exercise by project managers having rich experience with clinical trial methodologies. Timelines should be forecasted based on prior experience, study requirements and available resources, with acceptable limits of extending or shrinking under uncertain circumstances. Timelines may be affected by the following factors:

- Available resources
- Expertise and prior clinical research experience of sponsor, study site and CRO
- Treatment schedules and follow-up procedures
- Size and developmental phase of the trial
- Inclusion and exclusion criteria and overall design of the study
- Unexpected delay in regulatory review and approval
- Administrative issues (e.g. change of study monitor)

There may be other factors affecting the timeframe of clinical trial activities, which need to be identified while forecasting and controlling the timelines of clinical trial activities.

Developing the Time Plan for a Clinical Trial

1. Make a sequential list of activities to be accomplished starting from initiation up to final completion of the project. It is advisable to break larger activities into smaller tasks, provided all the tasks can be achieved individually.
2. Group these activities into three time segments for a clinical trial project, i.e. before study initiation, during the study, and after the study.
3. Do "critical path analysis" for all the activities.
   a. Analyze the prerequisites for activities and designate them either as "parallel activity" or "sequential activity". A parallel

activity is that which does not depend upon the completion of any other activity, whereas a sequential activity is one that depends on the completion of one or more other activities or can only be initiated after one or more other activities.

b. Forecast the approximate time log (or a range of time log) required to complete individual activities duly considering the element of future uncertainty.

4. Prepare a "Gant chart" for all activities of the clinical trial depicting the time of initiation, sequence and time log for each individual activity.

Below is given a format/design for planning and forecasting the timelines of various trial related activities. The time log considered here is an arbitrary value, and this design may not contain all the study-related activities of a typical clinical trial. However, it can be used to develop a time plan for the study. Time log required for study procedures depends on the duration of therapy, follow-up and rate of recruitment.

Critical Path Analysis

S.No.	Clinical Trial Activities	Time Log (months)	Nature of Activity
Before the study initiation			
1	Study design & protocol preparation	3	Initial activity
2	QA/QC system design	2	Sequential - 1
3	CRF and database preparation & validation	2	Sequential - 1
4	ICF & PIS preparation and translations	2	Sequential - 1
5	Printing of protocol, CRF, ICF, PIS	3	Sequential - 1, 3, 4
6	IP procurement and labeling management	3	Sequential - 1
7	Investigators and sites evaluation	3	Sequential - 1
8	Investigators and sites selection	2	Sequential - 7
9	Regulatory dossier, submission and approval	6	Sequential - 1, 3, 4, 8
10	IRB dossier, submission and approval	3	Sequential - 1, 3, 4, 8
11	CTRD preparation and registration	1	Sequential - 1, 8, 9
12	Investigators meeting	1	Sequential - 9, 10
13	IP, documents & other study material shipment	1	Sequential - 9, 10
14	Site training and study initiation	1	Sequential - 9, 10, 12, 13

Contd...

During study conduct			
1	Subjects screening and recruitment	These are ongoing activities and required time logs depend on rate of recruitment, duration of therapy, and follow-up	Initial activity
2	Study procedures (treatment, sample collection, clinical and lab investigations, follow-up etc)		Parallel
3	IP accountability management (receiving, dispensing, retrieval, returning and destruction)		Parallel
4	Source data & documents management		Parallel
5	CRF recording & management		Parallel
6	AE handling, reporting and management		Parallel
7	Periodic monitoring visits		Parallel
8	Data management (data entry, quality check, queries resolution)		Sequential - 7
9	Deviations/non-compliance handling		Parallel
10	Documentation of all communications		Parallel
11	Study files updation and management		Parallel
12	Interim analysis, if any	1	As per protocol
13	Trial safety evaluation	1	As per protocol
14	ASR preparation & submission	1	On stipulated timelines
15	Trial progress reports & submissions	1	On stipulated timelines
16	Interim audit and follow-up, if any	2	As per protocol
17	Interim inspection and follow-up, if any	2	If declared
After study completion			
1	EC and regulatory notification	1	Parallel
2	Study files finalization and management	2	Parallel
3	Data management (data entry, quality check, queries resolution, database lock)	2	Parallel
4	Trial audit and follow-up if any	2	As per protocol
5	Site close-out visits	1	Sequential - 2, 3, 4
6	Trial inspection, if any	2	If declared
7	Final analysis & results	3	Sequential -3
8	CSR preparation	2	Sequential - 7
9	Site, EC and regulatory submissions	1	Sequential - 8
10	Manuscript preparation and publication	4	Sequential - 8

Tentative Timelines: Before Study Initiation

Months / Activity	1	2	3	4	5	6	7	8	9	10	11	12	Onwards...
1													
2													
3													
4													
5													
6													
7													
8													
9													
10													
11													
12													
13													
14													

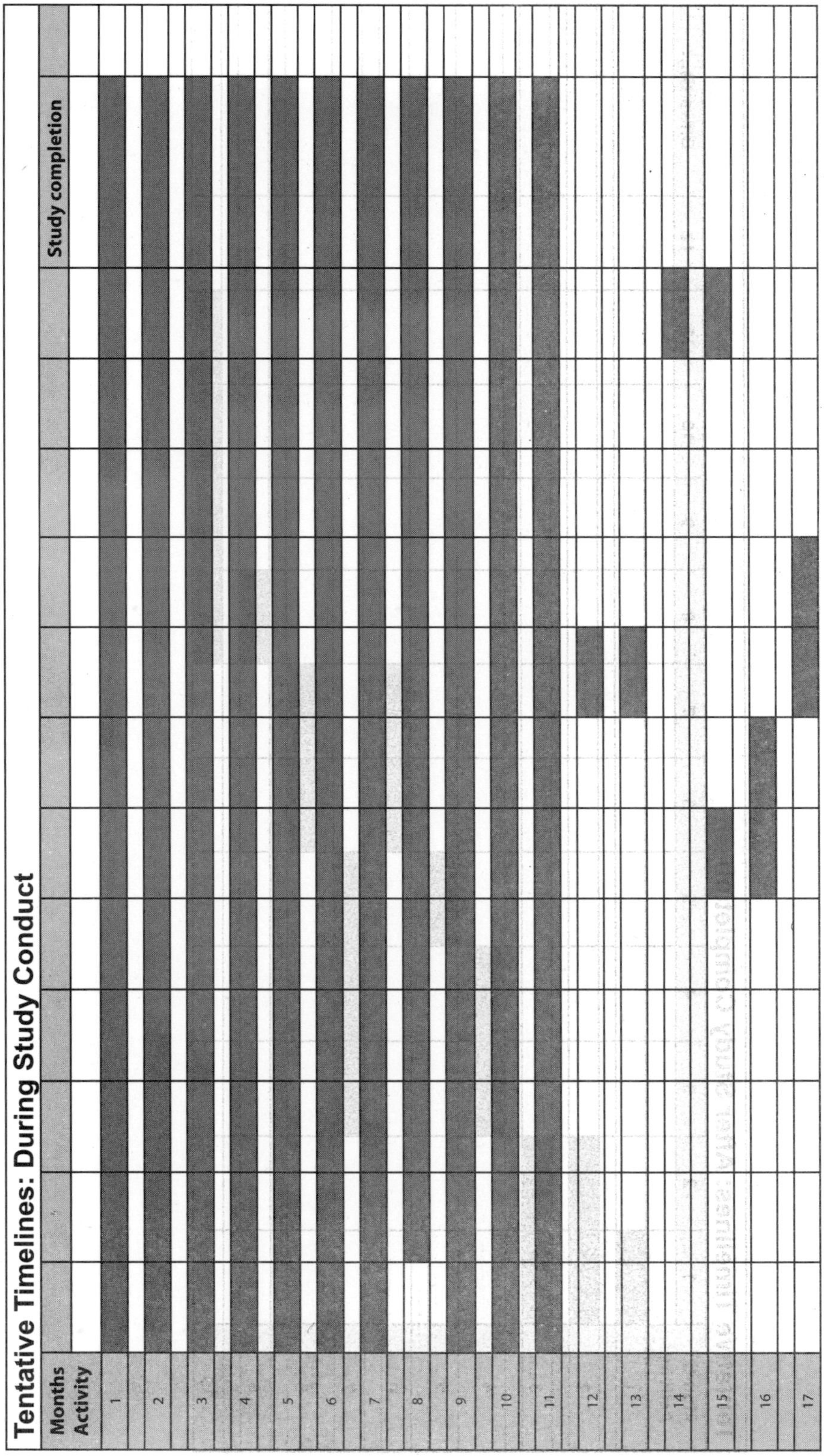
Tentative Timelines: During Study Conduct
Months
Activity
1
2
3
4
5
6
7
8
9
10
11
12
13
14
15
16
17
Study completion

Tentative Timelines: After Study Completion

Months / Activity	1	2	3	4	5	6	7	8	9	10	11	12	Onwards...
1													
2													
3													
4													
5													
6													
7													
8													
9													
10													

IMPLEMENTATION OF THE QUALITY SYSTEM

Effective implementation is one of the important parameters of a quality system to achieve the desired results. From the point of view of the sponsor, the following recommendations should be adopted for effective implementation of the quality system.

(a) Categorize the personnel involved in the clinical research project into three basic groups/parties, namely sponsor, vendors including CRO and other facilities if contracted/outsourced, and trial site.

(b) Make an exhaustive list of responsibilities (specified in detail) to be transferred to and carried out by them category-wise and individually. This listing will help identify "who is responsible for what" during the trial conduct.

(c) Appropriate training or instructions should be provided regarding their responsibilities, if required.

(d) Personnel strategies

- Create awareness regarding the importance of conducting clinical trials and subject safety, achieving satisfactory compliance in terms of monetary and time value for the sponsor, and the ill effects that the sponsor could come across due to non-compliance.
- Compliance is considered in the following categories:
  - Ethical compliance: It is related to the trial subject, and includes their safety, rights and wellbeing; maintaining confidentiality of identity (as per Declaration of Helsinki, GCP, Schedule Y and ICMR Code and applicable IRB).
  - Regulatory compliance: It is related to regulatory guidelines/requirements to be followed in conducting the trial procedures.
  - Sponsor compliance: It is related to approved protocol procedures and standard operating procedures.
- Make them understand the importance of their role in clinical development of a new drug which will help maintaining motivation, morale and enthusiasm.
  - Assign, explain and document the specific functions, tasks, responsibilities, and duties to be carried upon by every individual in the course of a clinical trial.

- Design appropriate training programs (on- and/or off-the-job) to improve their skills and knowledge for smooth functioning. Invite appropriate personnel with expertise in a particular area for training. Collect feedback from employees regarding the effectiveness of the training program and issues to be included for future training.

(e) If required, provide appropriate training/instructional materials on quality system, i.e. standard operating procedures to be followed, to all the parties involved in the clinical trial.

(f) To ensure effective completion of functions and duties by parties involved in the trial (e.g. CRO and trial site), all parties should sign on the legal documents/agreements containing all the pertinent sections/clauses (as described in regulations, sponsor-specific documents, protocol, etc) and describing specifically what, how, when, where and by whom the tasks, duties and functions are to be carried out.

(g) CRO and trial site

- Following the delegation of responsibilities, signed statements should be obtained and/or ensured.
- SOPs of CRO and trial site should be ensured and matched with sponsor and regulatory specific requirements.
- Facilities including IP storage, lab accreditation and certification, treatment equipment, and document archiving and retaining facilities should be ensured prior to the initiation of the trial.
- Adequate training/instructions should be provided prior to the initiation of the trial.

(h) A good communication and data handling system should be provided and designed by the sponsor or CRO (as per the agreement) to facilitate instant notification and discussion of problems any party may come across during the trial, thereby avoiding any delay in initiating appropriate corrective measures.

CONTROL AND EVALUATION OF THE QUALITY SYSTEM

Besides good planning, a trial needed to be constantly controlled and evaluated to avoid any deviation in its focus. Exercising and controlling all the activities according to predetermined standards is a milestone in the successful completion of a clinical trial.

Controlling and evaluation can be categorized into four parts for simplicity.

(a) Budgetary control

(b) Time control

(c) Recruitment and retention control

(d) Compliance control

Budgetary Control

Budgetary control implies controlling the monetary expenses for each activity individually and trial as a whole. The following recommendations can be considered.

1. The Project Manager should carefully allocate the funds for individual activities of the trial.
2. There should be adequate supervision on proper utilization of monetary resources for each activity; however discretion should be allowed among the staff to meet their obligation.
3. Wastages in resource utilization should be avoided as far as possible.
4. Periodic tracking of study-related expenses is required, which should be analyzed for each activity and study as a whole.
5. If any activity takes a significant deviation from the predetermined value, the project manager should analyze and try to find corrective measures.
6. The sponsor should continuously analyze trial activities in current situation and forecast the future costs so that suitable modifications can be made in prior budget of the project.

Time Control

Time control implies the controlling of time taken for accomplishment of each activity and the study as a whole. The project manager should periodically review the timelines of ongoing and accomplished activities to identify any delay or mismatch with timelines forecasted during the project planning stage. Factors responsible for time mismatch need to be identified. These factors can be classified as internal (Sponsor's control) or external (not in sponsor's control) factors. Suggesting and implementing the necessary corrective actions may be guided by the nature of influencing factor and need adequate prior clinical research experience.

Several digital tools are available nowadays, and may be considered for analyzing the timelines, identifying the limiting factors and preparing the corrective action. For example, "Gantt charts" are an excellent tool for organizing and scheduling the activities involved in a trial. Separate charts can be prepared for the three segments of a clinical trial, viz. before the trial, during the trial and after the trial. These time charts

- Help to plan tasks that need to be completed
- Give a basis for scheduling when tasks will be carried out and after which activity
- Allow to plan the allocation of resources needed to complete the activities and
- Help to monitor whether the project is running on schedule; if not, it helps develop the remedial action necessary to put it back on schedule.

Recruitment and Retention Control

Enrollment and retention of trial subjects are the two most important parameters on which resides the timeframe of the entire clinical study. These parameters should be analyzed before and during the clinical trial for the projection of timelines for the completion of the trial and for continuous tracking of the projected timeframe. If any difficulty arises, decision should be taken well before. Both Indian and ICH-GCP state that the investigator should be able to demonstrate the recruitment rate based on retrospective data and the sponsor should verify it at the time of investigator's selection and during the whole recruitment period of the trial and to come up with contingency plans if any mismatch arises.

The project manager should continuously analyze recruitment and retention parameters throughout the clinical study so that appropriate corrective actions can be initiated to keep the study timelines on track. It is advisable to decide the frequency of recruitment analysis and to organize periodic meetings with staff of trial sites to discover the root causes of poor recruitment or retention so that better strategies can be formulated and implemented. These parameters should be assessed both for individual trial sites and collectively for the whole trial. For the purpose of recruitment and retention analysis, the following definitions, methodology and estimations can be used for individual trial sites or the entire trial depending on the scope of analysis being done.

Definitions

1. Cumulative enrollment: Total number of subjects enrolled (on a cumulative basis) to the study/site, out of required/expected/projected enrollments, from the date of study/site initiation.
2. Percentage cumulative enrollment: Cumulative enrollment in percentages.
3. Current enrollment: Number of subjects enrolled (on current basis) to the study/site, out of required/expected/projected enrollments, from the date of previous enrollment analysis.
4. Percentage current enrollment: Current enrollment in percentages.
5. Enrollment rate: Number of subjects enrolled to the study/site per unit time. It can be estimated on cumulative or current basis.
6. Cumulative discontinuation: Total number of subjects discontinued (on a cumulative basis) including withdrawals, drop-outs and lost-to-follow-up, out of total enrollments, from the date of study/site initiation.
7. Percentage cumulative discontinuation: Cumulative discontinuation in percentages.
8. Current discontinuation: Number of subjects discontinued (on current basis) from the study/site out of total enrollments from the date of previous analysis.
9. Percentage current discontinuation: Current discontinuation in percentages.
10. Discontinuation rate: Number of subjects discontinued from the study/site per unit time. It can be estimated on cumulative or current basis.
11. Cumulative retention: Total number of subjects continuing or completed (on a cumulative basis) in the study/site out of total enrollments from the date of study/site initiation.
12. Percentage cumulative retention: Cumulative retention in percentages.

13. Current retention: Number of subjects either continuing or completed (on current basis) on the study/site out of total enrollments from the date of previous analysis.
14. Percentage current retention: Current retention in percentages.
15. Retention rate: Number of subjects either continuing or completed on the study/site per unit time. It can be estimated on cumulative or current basis.

Estimations

1. Cumulative enrollment (CE) = Total enrollments from the study or site initiation / Required or projected enrollments from the study or site initiation
2. % CE = CE × 100
3. Current enrollment (CrE) = Number of enrollments from the previous analysis / Required or projected enrollments from the previous analysis
4. % CrE = CrE × 100
5. Cumulative enrollment rate (CER) = Total enrollments from the study or site initiation / Time elapsed from the study or site initiation
6. Current enrollment rate (CrER) = Number of enrollments from the previous analysis / Time elapsed from the previous analysis
7. Cumulative discontinuation (CD) = Total discontinuations from the study or site initiation / Total enrollments from the study or site initiation
8. % CD = CD × 100
9. Current discontinuation (CrD) = Number of discontinuations from the previous analysis / Total enrollments from the previous analysis
10. % CrD = CrD × 100
11. Cumulative discontinuation rate (CDR) = Total discontinuations from the study or site initiation / Time elapsed from the study or site initiation
12. Current discontinuation rate (CrDR) = Number of discontinuations from the previous analysis / Time elapsed from the previous analysis

13. Cumulative retention (CR) = 1 – CD
14. % CR = 100 – % CD
15. Current retention (CrR) = 1 – CrD
16. % CrR = 100 – % CrD
17. Cumulative retention rate (CRR) = Total retentions from the study or site initiation / Time elapsed from the study or site initiation
18. Current retention rate (CrRR) = Number of retentions from the previous analysis / Time elapsed from the previous analysis

Analysis

The above estimations can be used to analyze:

1. Past and current situations of recruitment, discontinuation and retention
2. Trends (downward, upward or constant) of recruitment, discontinuation and retention
3. Mismatch, if any, between earlier projections and present situation and
4. Severity of mismatch by identifying the magnitude of gaps between earlier projections and present situation

Compliance Control

Compliance control involves maintaining the adherence of trial related activities with applicable regulatory guidelines, ethical guidelines and sponsor's requirements in order to achieve reliable and accurate data collection and safeguard the rights, safety and wellbeing of trial subjects. The following recommendations can be considered.

1. **Feedback Meetings**

   The sponsor should organize meetings at regular periodic intervals with all parties involved, i.e. sponsor, CRO, and trial site, to discuss critical aspects as below:

   - Training needs, if any, required
   - Difficulties in carrying out trial activities, if any
   - Probable remedial actions to be taken

2. **Assessment Tests**

   The sponsor may design and organize tests for personnel to assess their capabilities, knowledge and working behavior in order to project the compliance levels of trial activities. These assessment tests can be of the following types:

   (i) **Simulation Exercise** In this type of assessment, the personnel are assigned some cases and problems similar to those that arise in clinical trials, and their capabilities of handling those problems can be analyzed effectively.

   (ii) **Questionnaire Evaluation** The sponsor may design questionnaires to contain questions on specific problems and steps to be followed for performing these activities. Based on the findings, the sponsor can initiate actions to control the compliance level of the trial.

3. **Internal Audits**

   For effective measurement of compliance levels of trial activities, periodic internal audits may be an effective tool. Internal audits can also be merged with clinical trial audits as per the GCP standards. In order to obtain some meaningful actions to be taken for restoring the compliance, the sponsor can design audits with specifications of critical activities to be analyzed in detail by the auditors.

CONSTANT UPDATING OF THE QUALITY SYSTEM

The sponsor should update the quality system at periodic time intervals and whenever required. The sponsor should establish a quality system which meets the changing needs of clinical trials and regular upgrading of standards. The following recommendations can be considered.

- The sponsor should constantly organize feedback meetings to become aware of difficulties in the conduct of clinical trial as well as to suggest corrective actions to be initiated to meet the desired objectives.
- The sponsor should regularly identify and analyze the roots of problems and should try to select the most promising alternative course of action to avoid such problems.
- The sponsor or project manager may suggest modifications in standard operating procedures, which may lead to better

standardization and simplification of activities to be conducted. Hence the quality system should be reviewed and revised at regular intervals to incorporate necessary modifications.

- The personnel involved in clinical trials should be made aware of recent changes in regulations and guidelines pertaining to the clinical trial, and such changes should be incorporated into the quality system whenever necessary.

Summary of GCP

- Ethics are the product of morality and materialism. When morality is low, materialism is required to be high and vice versa.

> "Ethics = Morality × Materialism"

- Rights, safety and wellbeing of the participating subjects should be given utmost importance by all parties involved in the conduct of clinical research.

> "...Think...will it be acceptable
> By myself being a subject..."

- The principles of GCP are applicable to every individual involved in clinical research involving human subjects.

> "Every individual involved in clinical research is
> Bound to follow the principles of GCP."

- Any event, activity or process not documented is considered as "not happened". Adequate documentation of each trial related activity, function, process or event is a must for GCP implementation.

> "What remains after a trial...Documents...
> Which should reconstruct the trial
> and are the basis of approval."

> Life must be lived forwards, but can only be understood backwards...

- The same is true for clinical trials. A clinical trial can be reconstituted by person(s) not involved in trial conduct (e.g., regulatory authorities, IRB/IEC, auditor, etc.) only when all trial-related activities were documented properly.

> "...Document whatever you do...It should be in writing...
> If not documented...would be deemed as not happened."
> "Do what you write...Write what you do."

- Clinical trial data should be: ALCOA
  - Attributable
  - Legible
  - Contemporaneous
  - Original
  - Accurate

Closing Note

“Let us not follow
A path set by others;
Let us set a path
For others to follow.”

References

1. ICH Harmonised Tripartite Guideline: Guideline for Good Clinical Practice, E6(R1). Available at: http://www.ich.org/fileadmin/Public_Web_Site/ICH_Products/Guidelines/Efficacy/E6_R1/Step4/E6_R1__Guideline.pdf. Accessed April 2011.
2. Good Clinical Practices For Clinical Research In India: Schedule Y (Amended Version -2005). Available at: http://cdsco.nic.in/html/GCP1.html. Accessed April 2011.
3. ICH Harmonised Tripartite Guideline: General Considerations for Clinical Trials, E8. Available at: http://www.ich.org/fileadmin/Public_Web_Site/ICH_Products/Guidelines/Efficacy/E8/Step4/E8_Guideline.pdf. Accessed April 2011.
4. ICH Harmonised Tripartite Guideline: Clinical Safety Data Management-Definitions and Standards for Expedited Reporting, E2A. Available at: http://www.ich.org/fileadmin/Public_Web_Site/ICH_Products/Guidelines/Efficacy/E2A/Step4/E2A_Guideline.pdf. Accessed April 2011.
5. ICH Harmonised Tripartite Guideline: Statistical Principles for Clinical Trials, E9. Available at: http://www.ich.org/fileadmin/Public_Web_Site/ICH_Products/Guidelines/Efficacy/E9/Step4/E9_Guideline.pdf. Accessed April 2011.
6. Schedule Y, Drugs and Cosmetics Act and Rules. Available at: http://cdsco.nic.in/html/Drugs&CosmeticAct.pdf. Accessed April 2011.
7. S. Piantadosi, *Clinical Trials – A Methodological Perspective*, Second edition, John Wiley & Sons, Inc.

8. P.I. Good, *The Design and Conduct of Clinical Trials*, Second edition, John Wiley & Sons, Inc.
9. B.M. Mithal, *A Textbook of Forensic Pharmacy*, Tenth edition, Vallabh Prakashan.
10. D.R. Hutchinson, *How Drugs are Developed – A Practical Guide to Clinical Research*, Brookwood Booklets.
11. Understanding Clinical Trials. Available at: http://www.clinicaltrials.gov/ct2/info/understand. Accessed April 2011.
12. De, Minakshi, India Ideal Destination for Clinical Trials. *Current Science* 2005;l.89(4):25.
13. De, Minakshi, Clinical Trials in India. *Current Science* 2005; 89:597.
14. U.S. Food and Drug Administration (http://www.fda.gov).
15. The Drug Discovery, Development and Approval Process. Available at: http://www.fdareview.org/graphics/graph1.jpg. Accessed April 2011.
16. Human Experiments: A Chronology of Human Research by Vera Hassner Sharav. Available at: http://www.ahrp.org/history/chronology.php. Accessed April 2011.
17. Nazi Human Experimentation. Available at: http://en.wikipedia.org/wiki/Nazi_human_experimentation. Accessed April 2011.
18. Bioethic Chronology: A History of Broken Rules. Available at: http://www.sskrplaw.com/files/biochron1.pdf, Accessed April 2011.
19. Nuremberg Trials. Available at: http://en.wikipedia.org/wiki/Nuremberg_Trials. Accessed April 2011.
20. "Monster experiment" taught orphans to stutter. Available at: http://www.ahrp.org/infomail/0601/11.php. Accessed April 2011.
21. Count Two – War Crimes. Available at: http://www.ushmm.org/research/doctors/twoa.htm. Accessed April 2011.
22. Nazi Human Experimentations. Available at: http://individual.utoronto.ca/jarekg/Ravensbruck/Experiments.html. Accessed April 2011.
23. Nuremberg Principles. Available at: http://en.wikipedia.org/wiki/Nuremberg_Principles. Accessed April 2011.
24. Subsequent Nuremberg Trials. Available at: http://en.wikipedia.org/wiki/Subsequent_Nuremberg_Trials. Accessed April 2011.

25. WMA Declaration of Geneva. Available at: http://www.wma.net/en/30publications/10policies/g1/index.html. Accessed April 2011.
26. Declaration of Geneva. Available at: http://en.wikipedia.org/wiki/Declaration_of_Geneva. Accessed April 2011.
27. WMA International Code of Medical Ethics. Aavailable at: http://www.wma.net/en/30publications/10policies/c8/index.html. Accessed April 2011.
28. WMA Declaration of Helsinki – Ethical Principles for Medical Research Involving Human Subjects. Available at: http://www.wma.net/en/30publications/10policies/b3/index.html. Accessed April 2011.
29. Tuskegee Syphilis Study. Available at: http://www.brown.edu/Courses/Bio_160/Projects2000/Ethics/TUSKEGEESYPHILISSTUDY.html. Accessed April 2011.
30. The Belmont Report: Ethical Principles and Guidelines for the Protection of Human Subjects of Research. Available at: http://ohsr.od.nih.gov/guidelines/belmont.html. Accessed April 2011.
31. Nuremberg Code. Available at: http://ohsr.od.nih.gov/guidelines/nuremberg.html. Accessed April 2011.
32. Research Involving Persons with Mental Disorders that May Affect Decision Making Capacity. Available at: http://bioethics.georgetown.edu/nbac/capacity/TOC.htm. Accessed April 2011.
33. The History of the European Union. Available at http://europa.eu/abc/history/index_en.htm. Accessed April 2011.
34. History of ICH. Available at: http://www.ich.org/about/history.html. Accessed April 2011.
35. Organisation of ICH. Available at: http://www.ich.org/about/organisation-of-ich.html. Accessed April 2011.
36. Process of Harmonisation. Available at: http://www.ich.org/about/process-of-harmonisation.html. Accessed April 2011.
37. Glossary. Available at: http://www.ich.org/glossary.html. Accessed April 2011.
38. Advisory Committee on Human Radiation Experiments. Available at: http://www.gwu.edu/~nsarchiv/radiation/. Accessed April 2011.
39. Consort: Transparent Reporting of Trials. Available at: http://www.consort-statement.org/?o=1001. Accessed April 2011.

40. CDISC:Clinical Data Interchange Standards Consortium. Available at: http://www.cdisc.org/. Accessed April 2011.

41. Booming Clinical Trials Market in India. Available at: http://www.marketresearch.com/product/display.asp?productid=2066259. Accessed April 2011.

42. Clinical Trials in India. Available at: http://www.researchandmarkets.com/reportinfo.asp?report_id=591033. Accessed April 2011.

43. Brief History. Available at: http://osp.ua.edu/site/PRCO_History.html. Accessed April 2011.

44. Ethical Guidelines for Biomedical Research on Human Subjects – Indian Council of Medical Research. Available at: http://icmr.nic.in/ethical_guidelines.pdf. Accessed April 2011.

45. The Sulpha Elixir Tragedy. Available at: http://en.wikipedia.org/wiki/Elixir_Sulfanilamide_disaster. Accessed April 2011.

46. Significant Dates in U.S. Food and Drug Law history. Available at: http://www.fda.gov/AboutFDA/WhatWeDo/History/Milestones/ucm128305.htm. Accessed April 2011.

47. History. Available at: http://www.fda.gov/AboutFDA/WhatWe Do/History/default.htm. Accessed April 2011.

48. Milestones in U.S. Food and Drug Law History. Available at: http://www.fda.gov/AboutFDA/WhatWeDo/History/Milestones/default.htm. Accessed April 2011.

49. FDA's Origin & Functions. Available at: http://www.fda.gov/AboutFDA/WhatWeDo/History/Origin/default.htm, Accessed April 2011.

50. Food and Drug Administration. Available at: http://en.wikipedia.org/wiki/Food_and_Drug_Administration_(United_States)#History. Accessed April 2011.

51. European Medicines Agency. Available at: http://www.ema.europa.eu/ema/index.jsp?curl=pages/about_us/general/general_content_000235.jsp&murl=menus/about_us/about_us.jsp&mid=. Accessed April 2011.

52. Fraud and Misconduct In *Biomedical Research: Anil Aggrawal's Internet Journal of Forensic Medicine and Toxicology* 2004;5(1). Available at: http://www.indianjournals.com/ijor.aspx?target=ijor:aaijfmt&volume=5&issue=1&article=br-tb-006.

53. Clinical Trials Registry – India, National Institute of Medical

Statistics (ICMR). Available at: http://www.ctri.in/Clinicaltrials/index.jsp. Accessed April 2011.

54. Information Sheet Guidance for Sponsors, Clinical Investigators, and IRBs: Frequently Asked Questions – Statement of Investigator (Form FDA 1572). Available at: http://www.fda.gov/downloads/RegulatoryInformation/Guidances/UCM214282.pdf. Accessed April 2011.
55. Make Your Move: Taking Clinical Trials to the Best Location. Available at: http://www.atkearney.com/index.php/Publications/make-your-move.html. Accessed April 2011.
56. Drug Companies Cut Costs with Foreign Clinical Trials. New York Times. Available at: http://www.nytimes.com/2005/02/24/business/24clinic.html. Accessed April 2011.
57. W.G. Stough, F. Zannad, B. Pitt, et al., Globalization of Cardiovascular Clinical Research: The Balance between Meeting Medical Needs and Maintaining Scientific Standards. *Am Heart J* 2007;154:232-8.
58. C.W. Schmidt, Monitoring Research Overseas. *Modern Drug Discovery* 2001;4:25-6.
59. A. Bhatt, Evolution of Clinical Research: A History Before and Beyond James Lind. *Perspectives in Clinical Research* 2010;1(1):6-10.
60. J.P. Garnier, Rebuilding the R&D Engine in Big Pharma. *Harv Bus Rev* 2008;86:68-76.
61. S.W. Glickman, J.G. McHutchison, E.D. Peterson, et al., Ethical and Scientific Implications of the Globalization of Clinical Research. *N Engl J Med* 2009;360(8):816-823.